Nutrition and Endurance
Triathlon

Where Do I Begin?

Ironman Edition

Nutrition and Endurance

TRIATHLON

Where Do I Begin?

By Sheila Dean

MS, RD, LD/N, CDE

Published by Meyer & Meyer Sport

British Library Cataloguing in Publication Data
A catalogue record for this book is available from the British Library

Dean, Sheila:
Nutrition and Endurance – Triathlon
Where Do I Begin?
Oxford: Meyer & Meyer Sport (UK) Ltd., 2004
ISBN 1-84126-105-X

© 2004 by Meyer & Meyer Sport (UK) Ltd.
Aachen, Adelaide, Auckland, Budapest, Graz, Johannesburg,
Miami, Olten (CH), Oxford, Singapore, Toronto
Member of the World
Sports Publishers' Association (WSPA)
www.w-s-p-a.org
Printed and bound by: Gráficas, Santamaría, Spain
ISBN 1-84126-105-X
E-Mail: verlag@m-m-sports.com
www.m-m-sports.com

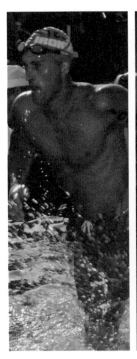
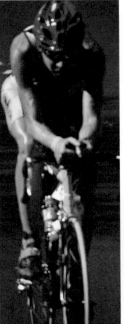
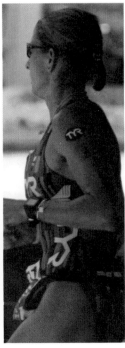

Contents

Part I – Ready, Set, Go!

Part II – Nutrition Basics

Part III – Get Supplement Savvy

Appendices

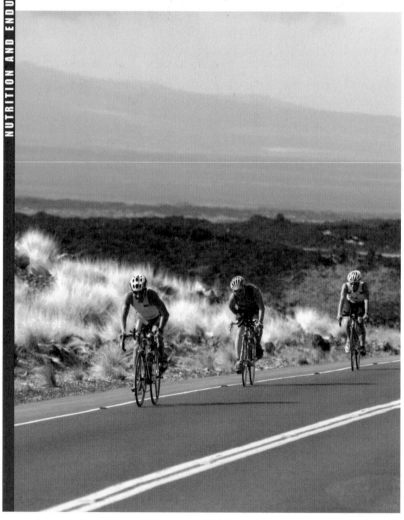

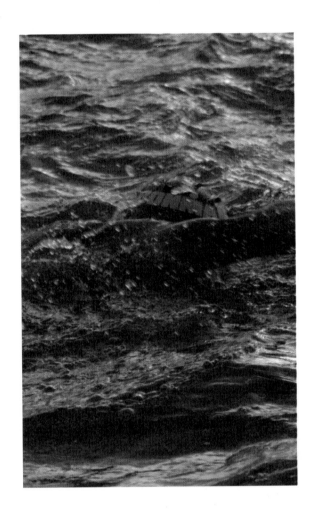

PART 1
Ready, Set, Go!

Acknowledgements

Many people have been involved in the creation of this book. I thank everyone equally, and here I wish to acknowledge a few.

First, thank you Thomas Stengel, of Meyer & Meyer publishing, for your direction, patience and encouragement throughout the entire book writing process. You are a pleasure to work with!

I am deeply indebted to Blair LaHaye and especially Ashley Mustard for all their time and effort in proofreading the book.

Thank you Tom "Doc" Manfredi, Ph.D and Linda Lamont, Ph.D, of the University of Rhode Island, for being more than just professors, but for inspiring me with your compassion, respect and firmness, to become a real scientist, writer and educator. Thank you for giving me the opportunity to not only help myself but, even better, "pass it forward." I am eternally grateful!

Thank you to registered dietitians, Christine Miller, MS, RD, LD, CDE and Jennifer Hutchinson, RD, LD, CSCS, and personal trainer, Eric Mabie for your gracious and prompt assistance with all my urgent questions.

Thank you to all my students, whose challenging questions have helped shape and mold this book.

Thank you to Billy Joon for your love and support! You are amazing. Thank you to my wonderful parents, Iraj and Faye and sister, Michele, for believing in me from day one. And of course, thank you little Emily and Nicholas, my heart and soul, for letting me know when it was time to take a break.

Finally, Thank you, Baha'u'llah, for making it happen.

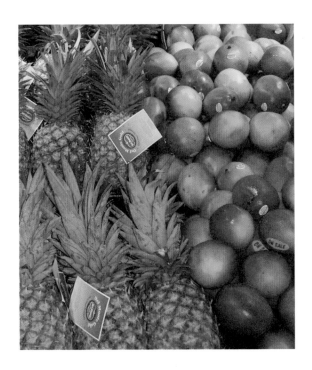

CHAPTER 1
Nutrition 101

In the busy pace of our modern lifestyle, athletes (whether a neophyte or an erudite) want the latest information on sports nutrition and they want it NOW! But with sensationalist media headlines, endless advertising, and growing Internet information, what is the athlete to believe? Clearly, the need for the qualified health professional to disseminate scientifically substantiated sports nutrition information is not just desirable, it's critical.

Think about it. If you wanted medical advice, you'd go to a physician. If you needed to know the law, you'd ask an attorney, if you had to do your taxes, you'd seek the assistance of an accountant. When it comes to nutrition, it's just as important that the information and advice needed is given by a qualified nutritionist/registered dietitian (R.D.). If you are thinking about entering the world of triathlon, or even your first 5K run, you will want to understand the primary factors that influence an athlete's performance. Of course, all serious athletes train diligently. The difference between the winner and the others rests with three main factors: their genes, their will to win and their diet. You can't do much about your genes, and the power of belief is nothing to scoff at, but more athletes are learning that your training diet is just as important for achieving maximal performance. If you are going to talk nutrition, you should know what the word means!

In the Beginning…

Nutrition is the science of how the body uses food, not the art of food and cooking. A nutrient is a chemical substance that supports cell growth, maintenance and repair. Just keep in mind though that a nutrient must meet all three criteria, not just one or the other. For example, alcohol would not qualify as a nutrient, as it interferes with the growth, maintenance, and repair of the body.

So what are they? Nutrition scientists have placed nutrients into six categories:

▲ Carbohydrates
▲ Fats
▲ Proteins
▲ Vitamins
▲ Minerals
▲ Water

Of these six nutrients, three contain calories and three do not. You may have already guessed that carbohydrates, fats and proteins contain calories. Think of calorie as a word that measures something, such as the word "dozen", which measures 12 of anything. In this case, calories measure the amount of heat produced when food is burned in your body cells.

In the nutrition science world, the word "calorie" and "energy" are synonymous; and only carbohydrates, fats and protein give you energy. The other three DO NOT. They do, however, act as "little helpers." Foods cannot be properly processed by the body without vitamins, minerals and water.

This is why vitamin/mineral manufacturers that tout their supplements as providing "energy" or "vigor" are very misleading. It is also the reason why a person could not go on a starvation diet and just pop a multivitamin to compensate for the absence of proper nutrition from food.

Here's the lowdown on the 6 nutrients.

Carbohydrates

Carbohydrates consist of three varieties. They are simple sugars, complex starches and fiber. Yes, fiber falls under this category.

Examples of different types of simple sugars are sucrose (table sugar), fructose (fruit sugar), and lactose (milk sugar). They are called simple because they are simple for your body to break down or digest. The simplest sugar is called glucose.

Examples of complex carbohydrates (starchy foods) are grains such as pasta, rice, potatoes, crackers, cereals, etc. Some vegetables are also starchy, like corn and peas. Both simple and complex carbohydrates provide 4 calories for every gram of it you eat. So, if a label says 1 slice of bread has 15 grams of carbohydrates, you would know that equaled 60 calories of carbohydrates (15 x 4 = 60). Ultimately, both types of carbohydrates get digested down into glucose (sugar). That's why we refer to the sugar in your blood as "blood glucose" or "blood sugars." The two are synonymous.

Where Does Fiber Fit into All of this?

Although fiber is considered a type of carbohydrate, it does not yield calories in the human body because we don't have the enzymes to break down fiber. It is true that normal intestinal bacteria can break down fiber a little, but basically, fiber is just calorie-free.

So what's all the hype about fiber and why have studies shown that a diet high in fiber has been associated with a lowered risk of heart disease, certain cancers, and an improved cholesterol level? First you should know that there are two types of fiber: soluble and insoluble. Oats, barley and pectins (the gummy substance in fruits like apples) are considered soluble fibers. That's the type of fiber that's related to a decreased risk of heart disease and for improved cholesterol levels. The proposed mechanism is that soluble fibers can "bind" to parts of cholesterol, which ends up getting excreted.

Insoluble fiber is found mainly in wheat bran and vegetable stems and leaves. This kind of fiber is related to a decreased risk for certain types of cancer like colon cancer. The general idea is that insoluble fibers "slough" off dead intestinal cells that are potentially carcinogenic (cancer-causing), allowing a new generation of healthy cells to grow.

Did you know that the brain only accepts glucose for fuel?

Fat

Lipids and triglycerides are just two fancy-sounding words that basically mean fat. There are also other "relatives" of fats called sterols and phospholipids. Examples are cholesterol and lecithin, respectively (Yes, lecithin is a type of fat). However, the majority of fats in foods are in the form of triglycerides.

There are different types of fats. Fats can either be:
1. saturated or
2. unsaturated.
If they are unsaturated then they can be further divided into:
a. monounsaturated or
b. polyunsaturated

The rule of thumb is that all animal fats are saturated. This includes any type of meat, poultry or fish, milkfat, butter... if it came from an animal and it has fat, it's saturated. Does this mean that all plant fats are unsaturated? NO, not all, but most. The exception to the rule are coconut oil and palm oil (known as the "tropical oils"), which are highly saturated also. It is these types of artery clogging fats that cause heart disease.

Examples of monounsaturated fats are canola oil and olive oil. These are the heart healthy fats. Examples of polyunsaturated fats are vegetables oils such as corn oil, sunflower oil, safflower oil. These fats are more neutral. They are not so bad but they are not so good.

Fats are only created equal when it comes to the number of calories per gram - nine. So whether you're using extra virgin olive oil on your tossed salad or you are using lard in your cooking, you always get the same number of calories. Of course, this can lead to weight gain if you eat too much. The effect on heart and artery health is what differentiates one fat from another.

The degree of saturation influences the firmness of fats at room temperature. The more saturated the fat is, the harder it will be at room temperature. Compare an oil, such as corn oil, to butter. The oil is liquid at room temperature because it is less saturated than butter.

Did you know that diseases of the heart and blood vessels, collectively known as cardiovascular diseases, are the single leading cause of death around the world today?

Protein

Many people associate proteins with meat, and although it is true that meat is primarily protein, there are many plant foods that are good sources of protein as well.

The building blocks of proteins are made up of structures called amino acids which combine together in many different variations. Imagine a string of beads of various colors and shapes. The beads are like the amino acids and the string is the protein. And these different strings, or proteins, have different functions in the body. Some are hormones, some are enzymes, muscle fibers, antibodies, neurotransmitters, organs... the list goes on. Similar to fats, there are also "essential amino acids" that can't be synthesized in the body. They must come from the diet. There are nine essential amino acids, compared to only two essential fatty acids. Protein contains 4 calories per gram, but your body prefers not to use it as a major source of energy. Instead the body gets its energy from fat and carbohydrates.

Did you know that excessive animal protein in the diet can increase your risk of osteoporosis?

Vitamins

In contrast to the three nutrients just discussed, vitamins do not provide energy or calories directly. Instead, vitamins act like "little helpers" because they help facilitate many metabolic reactions in the body. Vitamins activate the enzymes which are responsible for the break down and building of different nutrients. The claim that certain vitamins help provide energy refers to this indirect relationship.

The vitamins include A, B-complex, C, D, E, and K. They are usually referred to as water-soluble (includes B-complex and C) and fat-soluble (A,D,E,K). Water-soluble vitamins are generally excreted in urine if we consume them in quantities greater than our bodies need. As a result, people are usually able to take pretty high doses of B-complex and C without toxic effects. Fat-soluble vitamins, however, are not as readily excreted and instead are stored if taken in amounts greater than needed. So, taking very high doses, sometimes referred to as pharmacological doses, can be dangerous, particularly for vitamins A and D. Vitamins are easily destroyed by things like heat, light and oxygen.

Did you know that almost every action in the body requires the assistance of vitamins?

Minerals

Minerals, like vitamins, do not contain calories. However, unlike vitamins, minerals are indestructible. On the down-side, they can be bound by substances that make it difficult for the body to absorb them or may even leech out of food and get discarded with the cooking water. There are at least 16 different minerals that we know to be essential for the human body, but others are being studied to determine whether they play a significant role in human health. Some minerals can form salts that dissolve in water, such as sodium chloride, also known as table salt. Chapter 8 describes some of the more popular minerals, such as electrolytes, which can be especially important for the athlete.

Did you know that some minerals are needed in micrograms, an amount 1/1000 of a milligram, yet without it serious health problems could result?

Water

This is the most neglected nutrient – your body is about two-thirds water. It is absolutely indispensable and unlike food, we can't go without water for more than just a few days without suffering from serious dehydration or even death. In your body, water is the fluid in which all life processes occur.

Water imbalances can be devastating as water holds an impressive list of functions and its volume is tightly regulated. In fact, people who tend to retain water are usually those who are walking around dehydrated! The reason? If you are not drinking enough water on a regular basis, your body will hold on to water that it desperately needs for metabolic processes.

The solution? To lose water you've got to drink water. In other words, to relieve that uncomfortable bloated feeling, you've got give it what it needs - more water. The result is that your body will gladly release the extra water via the urine and you'll be feeling better and less sluggish in no time. The obvious dietary sources are water itself and other beverages, but nearly all foods also contain water. Most fruits and vegetables contain up to 95 percent water, while many meats and cheeses contain at least 50 percent water.

Putting it Together with the Food Guide Pyramid

Simply put, the Food Guide Pyramid is a graphic depiction of the basic food groups that should be included in our everyday diet. Its focus is to illustrate both individual serving sizes and total servings of foods from each of the food categories. Concepts of balance, variety and moderation have been "built in" to the recommendations of the food guide pyramid.

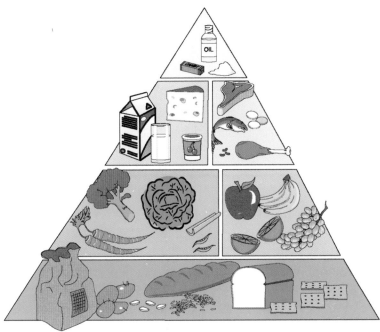

The base of the pyramid consists of carbohydrate-based foods and should be consumed most often, while the top of the pyramid represents fats and sugars which should be consumed sparingly. Specifically, it recommends 6-11 servings from the grain group, 3-5 servings from the vegetable group, 2-4 servings from the fruit group, 2-3 servings from the milk group, 2-3 servings from the meat, beans and nut group.

Eating the lower end number of servings will provide about 1600 calories and eating the higher end number of servings will provide about 2800 calories. The Food Guide Pyramid is not intended to replace special individual nutrient needs, nor is it appropriate for those who are in the disease-state.

Using the Food Guide Pyramid is a good starting point for meal planning. The major problem with the Food Guide Pyramid is that it doesn't show the importance of water. As usual, water is the most neglected nutrient, yet we couldn't live without it for more than a few days.

Evaluate Your Plate

A great way to get started on a healthy eating program is to first evaluate your plate. In other words, keeping a food journal of everything you eat for a few days or even a few weeks will give you a clear idea of what you really are putting in your mouth! Use the Daily Food Journal in the appendices to help you get started. Once you've recorded a few days' or weeks' worth, start looking for trends. Consider taking it to a registered dietitian who can assess it for you and give you a comprehensive report of what your diet looks like and how you can improve it to achieve your goals.

Did you know that only 1 cup of cooked rice counts as 2 servings from the grain group of the food guide pyramid?

Table 1
Calories provided for lower and upper end recommended servings of the Food Guide Pyramid

Food Group	Servings	
Grain	6	11
Vegetable	3	5
Fruit	2	4
Milk/Yogurt/Cheese	2	3
Meat/Beans/Nuts	2	3
Total Calories	1600	2800

NUTRITION AND ENDURANCE - TRIATHLON ••• 20

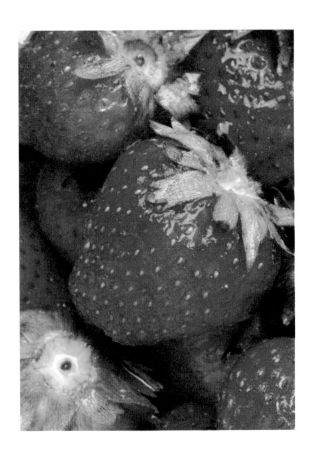

CHAPTER 2

The Basics of Healthy Eating

In order to transition from your current eating habits to eating like an athlete, it will take a bit of time and adjustment. But a great way to get started is by following these three key nutrition guidelines:

1. Eat frequently. Spread out your calories throughout the day. Frequently, people are in the habit of not eating much food throughout the day and get so hungry that dinner time that they can't stop eating. This is one of the best ways to get fat! I like to refer to this phenomenon as the "starve all day, stuff all night" syndrome. When you eat too much in the evening, it is almost natural to not feel so hungry in the morning, which perpetuates this cycle. You must understand that eating breakfast, lunch, dinner and even snacks throughout the day can make all the difference in the world. By eating small, frequent meals (not more than 4 hours without eating) this will help prevent overeating at meals. Avoid both "picking" at food or eating too much in one sitting. This will keep you feeling full all day. It will also keep your blood sugars more stable, thereby avoiding hunger pangs that cause cravings, irritability, low energy and headaches. Snacks can make or break the diet. Choose fresh fruit and vegetables with low or nonfat dairy products for a healthy carbohydrate and protein balance.

Examples of good snacks are:

▲ Part-skim mozzarella cheese strings

▲ Plain, nonfat yogurt with raw vegetables

▲ Flavored non- or low-fat yogurt topped with slivered almonds and seeds

▲ Fresh fruit and non- or low-fat cottage cheese

▲ Whole wheat crackers with natural peanut butter

▲ Pita bread with hummus

▲ Energy bars that are not very high in carbohydrates or protein, but rather have a balance of carbohydrate, protein and fat

2. Choose high fiber carbohydrates. To carb or not to carb! It's a popular question. There are many controversies that surround this subject. I'm convinced that carbohydrates are a very healthy part of the diet and to completely eliminate or drastically reduce these precious energy producing nutrients would be devastating to your energy levels and exercise performance. However, the trick is to choose foods containing carbo-hydrates that are also high in fiber and low in refined sugars. Fiber is a type of carbohydrate that slows down digestion and the rate at which starch and sugar in the food eventually becomes sugar in your bloodstream. When this happens your body will release insulin, a hormone to lower blood sugars more slowly, thereby preventing a sudden drop in blood sugars. This "balance" in blood sugars will prevent you from feeling as hungry and will reduce the cravings for food, ultimately leading to a healthier diet and possibly weight loss. Your total fiber intake should optimally be 20-25 grams daily. Choose high fiber cereals (that is, cereals with greater than 5 gms of dietary fiber), 100% WHOLE wheat breads, fresh fruits, fresh veggies, beans, whole wheat crackers and pasta. Look for the word WHOLE in the ingredients list.

3. Add protein to each meal. Like fiber, adding protein foods such as peanut butter, lean meat, eggs or egg whites, lean cheese, beans, and nuts will help to slow down digestion and stabilize blood sugars. Individuals are usually much more satisfied and less hungry if the meal was eaten with protein. For example, don't eat a slice of toast alone. Have it with natural peanut butter. Don't eat oatmeal alone. Eat it with an egg. Avoid eating pasta alone. Combine it with some meat such as lean chicken or fish. Your protein needs are about 0.8 – 1.0 gms/kg/day Ex: 150lbs = 68kg therefore, you need 54-68 grams of protein daily.
(Note: Simply divide your weight in pounds by 2.2 to get your weight in kilograms)

Did you know that you have to eat 3,500 excess calories in order to gain only 1 pound of fat, yet obesity is an official epidemic in the United States?

Label Lingo – What's in a Name?

Just the Facts, Please

The Bush administration approved legislation establishing the most extensive and consumer-oriented food labeling reform in the history of this country in 1997. The new Nutrition Facts labels, required by the U.S. Food and Drug Administration (FDA) on nearly all packaged foods, have made it much easier to choose foods in your overall diet to meet recommendations of the Dietary Guidelines for Americans and the Food Guide Pyramid. Nutrition Facts, however, differ from nutrition descriptions.

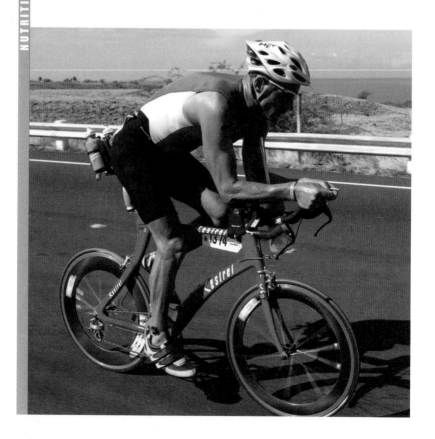

The Nutrition Facts panel specifically states the amount of nutrients and calories in food. Features on the Nutrition Facts panel include:

▲ Standardized serving size – is now based on how much people actually eat. For example, in the past if a product was high in fat, a company could make a serving size smaller to reduce its fat content. Now you don't have to compare a brand of soup that lists a serving size as 7.75 ounces with one that calls a serving 10.5 ounces.

▲ Calories - per single serving as well as calories from fat.

▲ % Daily Value – compares one serving to a 2,000 calorie diet. This does not reflect the percentage the product provides.

▲ Nutrient amounts – of the ones related to today's most important health issues.

▲ Daily footnote – that shows two calorie levels (2,000 and 2,500) and what the upper limit for total fat, saturated fat, cholesterol and sodium should be. The amounts listed for total carbohydrate and dietary fiber are target amounts rather than upper or lower limits.

▲ Calories per gram conversion – to show you how to determine total calories from fats, carbohydrate and protein. For instance, once you've figured total calories from carbohydrate, you can then figure the percent the product provides by simply dividing that number by the total calories per serving.

What the Food Labels Will Dish up For You

Nutrition descriptions or terms on a label are also FDA specified. These precise word definitions, issued by the FDA, also brought order to what had become a free-for-all on food labels. Categorized by nutrient, the following is a glossary of descriptive terms to help you make sense of the language of labels.

Fat and Cholesterol

Fat-free: less than 0.5 g of fat per serving (and no added fat or oil).
Non-fat: same as fat-free.
Skim: used in reference to a dairy product. It is synonymous with non-fat.
Low-fat: 3 g or less fat per serving.
Less fat: 25% less fat than the comparison food.
Reduced-fat: synonymous with less fat. So "reduced-fat" is a term that is used to compare the "new and improved" product with its original version. Foods termed "reduced fat" or "light in fat" can still have lots of fat. Reduced-fat *Better Cheddar* crackers, for example, still contain 6 grams of fat per serving and get 36% of their calories from fat.
Saturated fat-free: less than 0.5 g of saturated fat and 0.5 g of trans-fatty acids per serving.
Low saturated fat: 1 g or less saturated fat per serving.
Less saturated fat: 25% or less saturated fat than the comparison food.
Cholesterol-free: less than 2 mg cholesterol per serving and 2 g or less saturated fat per serving.
Low cholesterol: 20 mg or less cholesterol per serving and 2 g or less saturated fat per serving.
Less cholesterol: 25% less cholesterol than the comparison food (reflecting a reduction of at least 20 mg per serving), and 2 g or less saturated fat per serving.
Extra lean: less than 5 g of fat, 2 g of saturated fat, and 95 mg of cholesterol per serving and per 100 g of meat, poultry, and seafood.
Lean: less than 10 g of fat, 4.5 g of saturated fat, and 95 mg of cholesterol per serving and per 100 g of meat, poultry and seafood.
Light: 50% less fat than in the comparison food.

As a general guideline for meats, the lowest fat and fewest calories are found in skinless chicken breasts, skinless turkey breasts and pork or beef tenderloin. Also, "low-fat" is defined differently when it's on a milk carton. Dairies used to be permitted to keep this term for 2% milk, however, since January 1998, 2% milk is now required to be advertised as "reduced-fat", and not "low-fat" since it contains 5 grams of fat per serving. Keep in mind that milk contains 87% water, so even though we call it "2% milk", when you figure the percent of calories coming from fat, it is really 36% fat (5 grams/serving x 9 cals/gram = 45 fat calories and 45 ÷ 120 total cals = 36% fat). Since that is greater than 30%, it can't be called low-fat anymore. In other words, the product has to be less than 30% total fat to be considered a low-fat milk product.

Extra, Extra: An Update on Label Lingo!

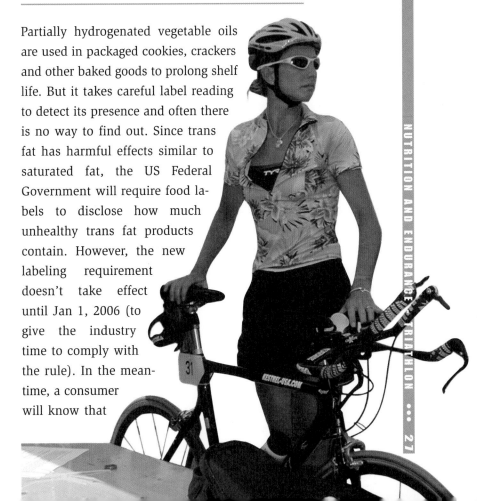

Partially hydrogenated vegetable oils are used in packaged cookies, crackers and other baked goods to prolong shelf life. But it takes careful label reading to detect its presence and often there is no way to find out. Since trans fat has harmful effects similar to saturated fat, the US Federal Government will require food labels to disclose how much unhealthy trans fat products contain. However, the new labeling requirement doesn't take effect until Jan 1, 2006 (to give the industry time to comply with the rule). In the meantime, a consumer will know that the product contains trans fats if the ingredients list includes "partially hydrogenated" oils. To figure out how much, consider this: If the label gives the amount of other fats (saturated, polyunsaturated and monounsaturated), add those figures together and subtract them from the amount of total fat. What remains should be the approximate amount of trans fat the product contains. For example, the nutrition label on Reduced Fat Wheat Thins crackers lists 4 grams total fat, 0.5 grams saturated fat, 0 grams polyunsat-

Table 2
Fat breakdown of common products

PRODUCT	SERVING SIZE	TOTAL FAT	SATURATED FAT	TRANS FAT
Biscuits (refrigerated dough)	55g	6.5g	1.5g	2.0g
Cake frosting (chocolate, ready-to-eat)	35	6.5	2.0	1.0
Cheese crackers	30	9.5	2.0	2.0
Chocolate chip cookies	30	8.0	2.0	3.0
Doughnuts (sugar or glazed)	55	14.0	3.5	4.0
French fries, frozen (before cooking)	85	8.5	1.5	3.0
Graham crackers	30	3.0	0.5	2.0
Popcorn, microwave	30	7.5	2.0	2.5
Pound cake	80	16.5	3.5	4.5
Snack crackers	30	7.0	1.0	2.5
Taco shells	30	8.0	1.5	2.5

urated fat, 1.5 grams monounsaturated fat. Subtracting them from the total fat content shows about 2 grams unaccounted for. It's probably 2 grams of trans fat.

The U.S. Department of Agriculture (USDA) lists several packaged foods that contain particularly high levels of trans fat, often more trans fat than saturated fat (see table). Each item represents a national brand, which the agency declines to name. For each packaged food category, the USDA gives the number of grams of total fat, saturated fat and trans fat per standard serving size. In most categories, the listed trans fat content is similar to that of other brands, but not always.

In December 1998, the FDA announced plans to clarify what it believed could and could not be written on dietary supplement labels. These regulations define more specifically the "structure/ function" claims that are permitted and the "disease" claims that are not. The proposal is consistent with recommendations made by the Commission on Dietary Supplement Labels, an independent panel mandated by the Dietary Supplement Health and Education Act (DSHEA) of 1994. Government and industry sources agree that greater clarity was needed because of the ambiguity of DSHEA. That act allowed dietary supplement manufacturers to make "structure/function" claims – claims that a product may affect the body's structure or functioning – but prohibited claims that a product could treat, diagnose, cure or prevent a disease. The proposal accepts DSHEA's distinction between "disease" and "structure/ function" claims, but defines it in greater detail and gives numerous examples to make its points:

▲ Products can't pretend to be in a disease-fighting drug class. For example "antidepressant" cannot be used, but "energizer" can.
▲ A manufacturer cannot claim "a role in the body's response to a disease."

▲ The phrase "supports the body's ability to resist infection" is forbidden but "supports the immune system" (a "normal body function") is allowed.

Energy

Calorie-free: fewer than 5 calories per serving.
Light: one-third fewer calories than the comparison food.
Low-calorie: 40 calories or less per serving.
Reduced-calorie: at least 25 % fewer calories per serving than the comparison food.

Carbohydrates: Fiber and Sugar

High-fiber: 5 g or more fiber per serving; a high fiber claim made on a food that contains more than 3 g fat per serving and per 100 g of food must also declare total fat.
Sugar-free: less than 0.5 g of sugar per serving.
Wheat: You can't assume that "wheat", "stone ground wheat", "natural wheat" bread or even bread with "natural whole-grain goodness" is whole-wheat bread. If whole-wheat is not the first ingredient on the list, it's not whole-wheat.
Other Carbohydrates: the resulting value after subtracting the dietary fiber, sugars, and sugar alcohols, (if sugar alcohols are declared) from the total carbohydrate.

More on Sugar – Sweet by Any Name

As a nation, Americans consume more sugar than any other food additive – over 125 pounds per person each year! Unfortunately, this excess sugar consumption can lead to both tooth decay and obesity. Many of us believe some sugars are better for us than others, but the fact is sugar – sucrose, glucose, fructose, lactose, dextrose and all of the "oses" – have little or no nutritive value. In fact, the only thing sugar offers us is 4 calories per gram. To help cut down your intake of sugar, it helps to know the various names for sugar and to read food labels carefully for hidden sources of sugar.

Common Sugars

Check food labels for these common types of "sugar." (When manufacturers list "sugar", they are referring to sucrose only).

Sucrose: common table sugar – refined, raw, turbinado, brown, molasses and powdered.

Lactose or "milk" sugar: occurs naturally in milk products.

Total invert sugar: a mixture of glucose and fructose sold only in liquid form.

Fructose (or levulose): in its natural state is the sugar found in fresh fruit and honey. It is also made commercially from corn sugar.

Corn syrup: produced by the action of enzymes or acids in corn-starch (High fructose corn syrup is derived from corn).

Dextrose (or glucose): the simplest form of sugar. All carbohydrates in the body break down into glucose.

Maltose is manufactured from starch.

Sugar Alcohols: sugar-like compounds derived from fruit or commercially produced from dextrose. Often the weight conscious consume "diet cookies" believing that these cookies are calorie-free or very low in fat and calories. The truth is that neither is true. "Diet cookies" simply means that instead of using the traditional sugar (or sucrose) in the product, a form of sugar called a sugar-alcohol (usually in the form of sorbitol) is used. The problem is that sorbitol yields almost as many calories as regular sugar (3 cals/gm for sorbitol versus 4 cals/gm for regular sugar). It's just not absorbed into the bloodstream as quickly as sucrose, so diabetics can enjoy these types of products. In addition, eating large amounts of sorbitol or other sugar alcohols may produce abdominal cramps, bloating and diarrhea. Sugar alcohols also don't promote dental caries, so it's often seen in "sugarless" gums or sugar free mints. Again, the gum and mints are not calorie-free; rather a different type of sugar is being used. Other types of sugar alcohols include mannitol, xylitol, malitol, isomalt, lactitol and maltitol.

Sugar-free or sugarless: although these foods can't contain sucrose (table sugar), they can have other sweeteners, including honey, corn syrup, fructose, sorbitol or mannitol. And sometimes these ingredients can make a food just as high in calories. If the food isn't low in calories, it must somehow say that it is not a reduced-calorie food. Sugar-free candies and gum, for example, might read "useful only in not promoting tooth decay".

Hidden Sugars

Because of our love of sweets, food manufacturers often use added sugars to make commercial foods more appealing to our palates. Even "non-sweet" foods like ketchup, salad dressings, breads, and luncheon meats often contain added sugars. Before you place an item in your shopping cart, check the label for any of the above-mentioned sugars. Be sure to read the entire label since manufacturers are allowed to list the various types of sugar separately. For instance, a popular snack cracker lists both sugar and high fructose corn syrup among its contents, while a butter-topped wheat bread contains sugar, honey, and corn syrup as added ingredients.

Sodium

Sodium-free and salt-free: less than 5 mg of sodium per serving.
Low sodium: 140 mg or less per serving.
Light: a low-calorie, low-fat food with a 50% reduction in sodium.

Light in sodium: 50% or less sodium than the comparison food.

Very low sodium: 35 mg or less per serving.

Unsalted, salt-free, no salt, no added salt, without added salt: although all these terms mean that no salt was added during processing, the food could have significant levels of sodium, either naturally or from substances added for preservation, leavening, or other purposes. Check the list of ingredients for monosodium glutamate (MSG), sodium bicarbonate, and sodium saccharin.

Other General Terms

Free: an amount so little that it is considered "nutritionally trivial." Synonyms include "without," "no" and "zero." Many make such a claim that a food does not contain a nutrient naturally, but only as it applies to all similar foods (for example, "raisins, a fat-free food").

Healthy: a food that is low in fat, saturated fat, cholesterol and sodium and that contains at least 10% of the Daily Values for vitamin A, vitamin C, iron, calcium, protein, or fiber.

High: 20% or more of the Daily Value for a given nutrient per serving; synonyms include "rich in" or " excellent source."

Less: at least 25% less of a given nutrient or calories than the comparison food; synonyms include "fewer" and "reduced."

Light or lite: any use of the term must specify what it is referring to (for example, "light in color" or "light in texture").

Low: an amount that would allow frequent consumption of a food without exceeding the Daily Value for the nutrient. A food that is naturally low in a nutrient may make such a claim, but only as it applies to all similar foods (for example, "fresh broccoli, a low-sodium food); synonyms include "little," "few" and "low source of."

More: at least 10% more of the Daily Value for a given nutrient than the comparison food; synonyms include "added."

Good source of, contains, or provides: product provides between 10 and 19% of the Daily Value for a given nutrient per serving.

Common Food Measurements

Gram (g): a unit of weight.

Milligram (mg): 1/1000 of a gram.

Microgram (mcg): 1/1000 of a milligram (1 millionth of a gram).

Teaspoon (tsp): contains 5 g, 5 cc (cubic centimeters) or 5 mL (milliliters).

Tablespoon (Tbsp): 15 grams or 3 teaspoons.

Ounce (oz): 30 grams or 2 tablespoons.

Cup (c): 8 ounces (oz.)

Sometimes other terms are used to define the contents of the food. For example:

Imitation food: a food that may be substituted for and resembles another food. It is nutritionally inferior with respect to vitamin, mineral or protein content.

Substitute food: a food that is designed to replace another.

Fresh: food in its raw state. The term can't be used on food that has been frozen, heated, or contains preservatives.

Fresh frozen: food that is quickly frozen while very fresh.

Homogenized: a process of breaking up and separating milk fat. This makes the texture of milk smooth and uniform.

Pasteurized: process of heating foods, such as raw milk and raw eggs, to a temperature high enough to destroy bacteria and deactivate most enzymes that cause spoilage.

Ultra pasteurized: process of heating food to a temperature higher than pasteurization. This extends the time it can be stored in the refrigerator or on the shelf.

UHT (Ultra High Temperature): process similar to ultra

pasteurization. With high heat and sterilized containers, food can be stored unopened without refrigeration for up to three months. Once opened, it needs refrigeration.

Diet or dietetic: Unless the label states otherwise, diet and dietetic foods that fall under the jurisdiction of the FDA must meet the same requirements as "low-calorie" or "light" foods. That is, they must contain no more than 40 calories per serving or have at least one-third fewer calories than the regular product. But read carefully – labels on such products as dietetic breadsticks and cookies may show that they are low in sodium only, not in calories.

Enriched or fortified: The product contains added vitamins, minerals or protein. If so, the "per serving" amounts of nutrients must be given in addition to the list of nutrients.

Good vs. Choice beef: Although most consumers shy away from beef that is labeled "good" because they think it is inferior to "choice" or "prime," good beef is actually leaner. It may be a little tougher, but it is more nutritious per calorie than either choice or prime beef.

Natural: Although most of us assume a certain level of purity or safety from a "natural" food, there are no guarantees that we're getting any such thing unless it's a meat or poultry product. That's because the FDA and the Federal Trade Commission (which oversees advertising) STILL do not have any regulations regarding the word "natural," while the meat-controlling USDA does. "Natural" on meat and poultry means that there are no artificial flavors, colors, preservatives, or synthetic ingredients of any kind, and that the food and its ingredients are not more than "minimally processed." The term "natural" on any other foods, such as baked goods, beverages, or processed foods doesn't have to mean anything at all.

Naturally flavored: the FDA requires that the flavoring in a "naturally flavored" product be the essential oil, extract, or other derivative of a juice, spice, herb, root, leaf, or other natural source. It does not guarantee that there are no artificial colors, preservatives, or other additives.

Bottled: as in "bottled water" is just that; water that's been put in a clear bottle. There are presently no fast and hard rules requiring bottled water manufacturers to do anything special to their water. Still, most agree that bottled water does taste better than tap water. Best bet: if the budget allows, consider installing a water purifying treatment system in your home such as a combination of activated carbon and reverse osmosis, two methods of contaminant removal. If not, stick with the cheapest brand of purified water you can find.

Juicing up on Fruit Juice Terminology

The good ol' days where drinking a cup of juice didn't require a professional nutritionist to help you sort out the real thing from juice imposters are, simply put, gone. With the variety of juice and juice drinks available you may wonder if products that are labeled "100% fruit juice" are nutritionally different from other types of juice beverages. This helpful mini-glossary of fruit juice related terms will give you a quick splash of juicy information.

Naturally sweetened: the FDA does not have a regulation regarding this term. But many manufacturers use it when they sweeten with a fruit or juice rather than with sugar.

100% pure fruit juice: juice that has no added water or sugar. It is not made from concentrate. While it may not have added vitamin C as other juice drinks do, it does have other naturally occurring nutrients such as folic acid, which are often lacking in juice beverages.

Full-strength juice, single-strength juice or reconstituted juice: all synonomous terms that mean non-diluted juice.

Juice beverage: juice that is mainly fruit juice but may have some water, added sugar or coloring. Juice beverages are often fortified with up to 100% of the RDI for vitamin C (60 mg).

Juice drink: a beverage that is mainly water, sugar and a little juice for flavoring. Products labeled as "ade", or "juice cocktail drink" fall under this category.

Fruit flavored drinks: beverages that resemble a fruit or vegetable juice in color and/or flavor, which contain some of the natural juice, but are less than 100 percent juice. They must be labeled to clearly state the juice content. This federal regulation applies to all diluted fruit or vegetable juice beverages in interstate commerce.

Development of the flavoring and coloring industry has made possible a wide range of processed beverages that are classed as soft drinks, whether carbonated or not. Noncarbonated fruit-flavored beverages that are in concentrated, dehydrated, powdered, or other forms, and which contain no natural fruit or vegetable juice, are often identified with a coin name; however, the products must include a statement on the label that no XY juice is included, with XY being the juice represented or implied.

Pass the Cheese, Please

Just because the production of cheese was used more than 4000 years ago, it doesn't mean understanding the way cheese is produced today is any easier. One look at this list and you'll see why:

Natural Versus Process

Cheese made directly from the curd of milk and not reprocessed or blended is known as natural cheese. Some of the natural cheeses are made from unpasteurized milk. Process cheese is made from natural cheese that has undergone additional steps, such as pasteurization. Other ingredients are often added for flavoring, a softer texture, and longer shelf life.

Types of Process and Other Cheese

Pasteurized Process Cheese: made by grinding, blending and heating one or more natural cheeses. An emulsifier also is added to it. It melts smoothly when heated.

Pasteurized Process Cheese Food: made the same way as pasteurized process cheese, but other dairy ingredients may be added. The process cheese food has more moisture and less fat than process cheese.

Pasteurized Process Cheese Spread: lower in fat and higher in moisture than pasteurized process cheese food. It is spreadable at room temperature.

Cold-Pack Cheese: made by grinding and mixing one or more natural cheeses. It is not heated during processing. It also is known as club cheese. Cold-pack cheese can be smoked, and other ingredients, including spices and other flavorings, may be added.

Cold-Pack Cheese Food: made the same way as cold-pack cheese except other dairy ingredients are added. Other possible additions include spices or flavorings, artificial colors and sweeteners.

Imitation Cheese: a product must be called an imitation cheese if it does not meet the government standards of the product it is imitating. Often vegetable oil is substituted for the milkfat. Some imitation cheese may melt differently than their counterparts, so you may want to do a little experimenting if you are going to cook with them.

Did you know that eating regular peanut butter (as opposed to natural peanut butter) is just as unhealthy for your heart as eating pure lard (animal fat) because of all the hydrogenated fats it contains?

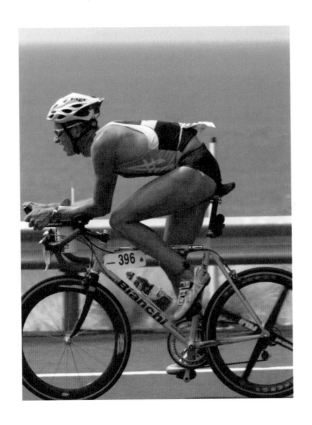

CHAPTER 3

Exercise Training 101

Death and taxes. Two things we all inevitably have to face at some point in our lives. You may as well add exercise to that list. Because no matter what anybody or any book ever tells you, there are no shortcuts, no secret formulas or magic ratios. You can't avoid exercise and still be serious about your health and fitness.

Why Exercise?

If you've never really exercised before, it may not start off being this euphoric experience that many claim it to be. It may even feel downright weird and uncomfortable to experience an elevated heart rate and all that sweat! The popular saying "no pain, no gain" is really quite inappropriate in this context. Exercise should not hurt. If it does, you should thank your body for recognizing that something is not right, and you should either slow down or just stop.

The fact is, our bodies were made to move. And it's a good thing too, because every drop of perspiration is a welcome antidote to the obesity epidemic that plagues the nation. You don't need to be an Olympic athlete, a marathon runner or even go to the gym every day to reap the benefits of exercise. What you do need is a little planning and consistency, and you'll find that exercise not only helps you lose weight – it can help you keep those pounds off for the long haul. Here's why:

▲ Regular exercise helps regulate your appetite.

▲ Regular exercise raises your energy level – so you're more likely to have the kind of active lifestyle that burns more calories.

▲ Exercise relieves tension – so you're less likely to eat to control stress.

▲ As you begin to exercise, you gradually build more muscle in your body and use up stored fat.

▲ As you build muscle and lose fat, you not only lose pounds, you look firmer and more toned.

▲ Regular exercise enables us to feel better about ourselves and more in control of our lives. These positive feelings are important predictors of weight management success.

▲ Exercise stimulates the immune system to significantly slow down the aging process. The converse is also true: inactivity speeds up human decline.

Although the benefits are clearly not limited to the ones I've just listed, one thing is certain: Exercise is medicine. "Medical fitness" proves that no single drug can out-do the impressive list of benefits that exercise provides. As you can see from this list, the main benefits of exercise have to do with maintaining and improving health. For those whose exercise habits are born out of their incessant drive for cosmetic beauty, just remember this: narrowly focused goals lead to narrowly focused solutions. When the desire to exercise is for achieving overall health, cosmetic beauty will automatically follow. Beautiful, isn't it?

Types of Exercise

There are generally three types of exercise. These are:

1. Aerobic exercise – the word "aerobic" means with oxygen. These exercises use large muscle groups, such as those of the legs, in some rhythmic fashion for a sustained period of time.

   For example, walking, jogging, biking, aerobic dance, step aerobics, etc. are all aerobic exercises. They all require the larger muscles of the body, can be done with a rhythmic pace and can be done for at least 15 minutes. So what does oxygen have to do with all of this? Well, because these exercises are done at lower intensities than say, sprinting, your body will need to find an energy source that can fuel itself for a longer period of time to do these exercises. The fuel of choice? FAT! And in order for fat to be used as fuel in the body, your cells need plenty of oxygen in them to burn fat efficiently. However, as important as aerobic or "cardio" exercise is, it does not increase resting metabolic rate. That is, the calories you burn from this type of exercise are really only achieved while you are actually exercising. According to the University of Florida's College of Health and Human Performance, there is no significant "after burn" or enhanced metabolic rate

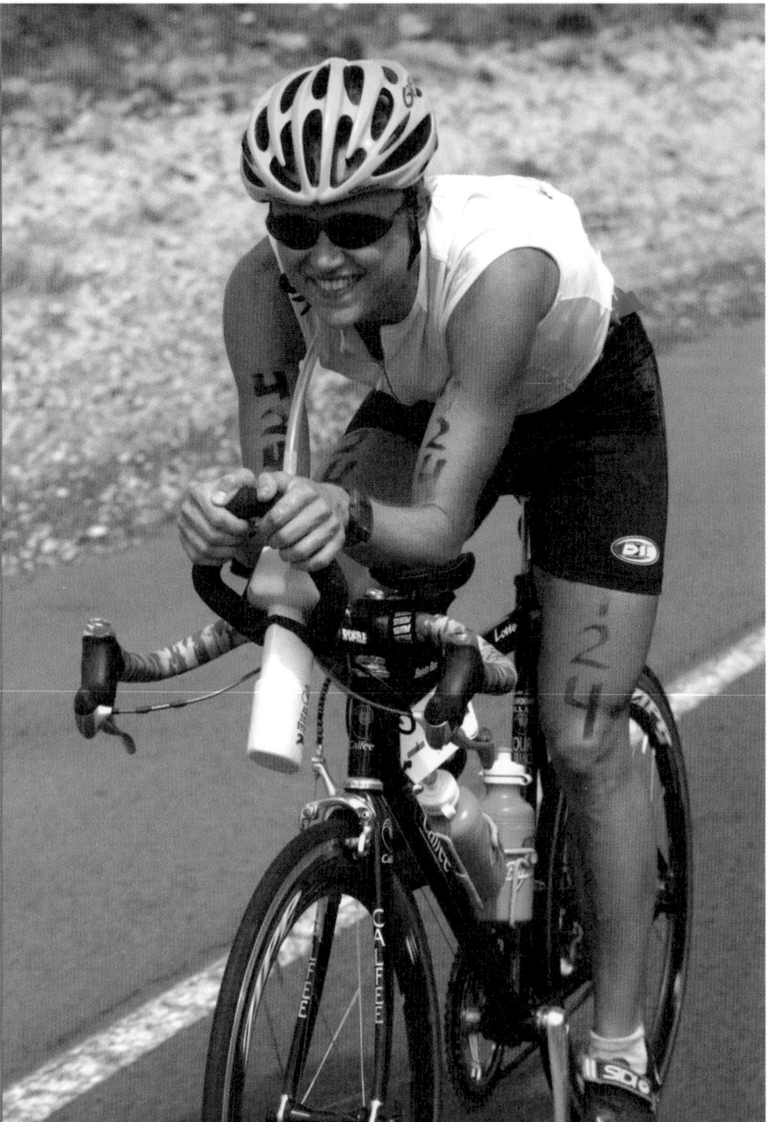

hours after you exercise aerobically. This is one of the very misunderstood aspects of exercise in general. As you will see with anaerobic or strength training, the story is quite different!

2. Anaerobic exercise/muscle strengthening – insert the letters "an" in front of the word aerobic and now it means without oxygen. Since oxygen is required for fat to be used as a fuel, it makes sense that fat is not the energy source of choice to fuel your body when performing fast, high-intensity exercises like sprinting. Stop-and-start type exercises also fall into this category, so activities like tennis and weight lifting tend to be considered more anaerobic in nature.

One of the many advantages of strength training is that when you increase the size and strength of your muscles, you are automatically increasing your metabolism. The two are directly proportional, so if you lose precious lean muscle mass, your metabolism slows down as well. The bottom line is that increasing the amount of muscle mass on your body will increase your metabolism, which can lead to weight loss. Why? Your body's skeletal muscle is a very "expensive" tissue. It takes a lot of fuel, or calories whereas fat tissue requires very little energy to function. In addition, anaerobic exercise makes you stronger, which can improve your ability to be physically active. Think about it. What is usually the limiting factor for individuals who claim that they can't move around much, or complain of aches and pain? Their level of STRENGTH or lack thereof. Unfortunately, clinicians too often do not prescribe progressive resistance or strength training to their patients for fear of thinking that there may be some inherent danger.

Another area of confusion is that people think that if you do a bunch of abdominal crunches or leg lifts, part of your body will slim down. Unfortunately, there is no such thing as spot reducing! If you do a hundred abdominal crunches every night for months, you may have abdominal muscles that are hard as a rock, but you'll still have a layer of fat (or several layers for that matter) on top! Muscle tissue and fat tissue are two different things. Strengthening the muscle will not magically melt away fat. If this were the case, then chewing gum would melt the fat off of your cheeks! According to Katch, Katch & McArdles' *Essentials of Exercise Physiology*, in order for a muscle to grow, it has to be actively exercised. YOU have to do the contracting of the muscle. It can't be contracted or exercised for you. No amount of jiggling, wiggling, or massaging of muscles will make them grow any bigger. Also, this type of passive exercise won't make fat disappear.

3. Stretching/flexibility – probably the most neglected type of exercise, yet one of the most important, is stretching. Stretching is not only an excellent way of improving your flexibility; it can also decrease your risk of all sorts of injuries, especially lower back injury, shin splints, and achy joints.

Before you begin stretching, make sure you do some kind of easy warm-up like walking or a slow ride on a stationary bike for 5-7 minutes. Once the blood is flowing, you're ready to stretch.

A common mistake people make when stretching is they think they must bounce to get a good stretch. For example, if you want to stretch your hamstrings (the back of your legs), you lift your leg up onto a chair or step and your reach for your toes. That's where you should just hold your stretch in a static fashion. No bouncing please! Why? Bouncing while stretching will actually do the opposite. Instead of trying to elongate the muscle, you are really making it contract more by bouncing!

The second common mistake is that after a workout, people just kind of stop without an adequate cool down and stretch. The next day, they are complaining that they can't exercise because they are too sore! If you're going to spend significant time exercising and contracting your muscles, they deserve to be stretched out for just a few minutes.

The cool down also helps remove metabolic waste products (that are often the cause of next-day soreness) that may have accumulated during exercise.

Now that you are convinced you need to exercise and the benefits are countless, how do you come up with an "exercise prescription?" Read on.

F.I.T.T. is an acronym that helps us come up with an exercise regimen. It stands for:

F – Frequency of exercise
I – Intensity of exercise
T – Time or Duration
T – Type of exercise

The American College of Sports Medicine (ACSM) is a highly respected organization that uses scientific research to create guidelines for exercise science and sports medicine. In a previous position statement, they claim that to achieve health benefits, one must exercise 3-5 days per week, at an intensity of 50-75% of his/her maximum heart rate, for 30-45 consecutive minutes per day.

Common "Training Diet" Mistakes

Practice makes perfect. You train over and over again so that on the day of your competition you are as prepared as you can be to win that race. Well, why not take that attitude with your training diet as well? After all, how can you compete at your best if you don't train at your best? And how can you train at your best if you're not fueled at your best? Here are a few examples of common mistakes to avoid in order to maximize your pre, during and post workout meals.

1. **Magic Foods.** Do you have that special "magic" food that seems to work for you when you're training? If so, don't assume that you'll have it the day you compete. Either bring it with you or make sure you have an alternative "magic" food that you can fall back on.

2. **Hydration.** Make sure that if you drink lots of water while you are training, you have access to water during your competition. If not, you may be left overly dehydrated and that's enough to impair your ability to compete. The opposite holds true also: if you're not accustomed to drinking plenty of water during training, then doing so on the day of the event will only leave you feeling bloated and uncomfortable. When training, practice eating and drinking the way you anticipate for the day of your competition. You don't want any unwelcome surprises the day of your event! Be careful!

3. **Avoid eating sweets** 15-45 minutes prior to exercise, especially if you know you are sugar-sensitive. An individual who is sugar-sensitive may experience symptoms like dizziness, fatigue or lightheadedness during exercise if they eat or drink sugary products. This is due to a rebound effect where blood sugars actually dip too low. In general, however, sugar is really not the main problem. The real problem is not eating enough at breakfast and lunch. Eating small frequent meals throughout the day is by far one of the best ways to prevent hunger (which results in overeating or choosing unhealthy "empty calories" for a quick fix). If you insist on eating a large meal, at least do so during the day. One nutritionist I know tells her clients to "fuel by day, diet by night".

4. **Choose nutrient-dense foods.** If you have a hard time getting fruits and vegetables in your training diet, don't waste your calories on those that don't offer many nutrients, such as grapes or iceberg lettuce. Instead choose the ones that'll give you the most nutrients for the least calories. Examples of fruits include oranges, grapefruit, bananas, melon, strawberries, and kiwi. Examples of vegetables include broccoli, peppers, spinach, tomato, carrots and squash. The rule of thumb is the darker the vegetable the better!

5. **Plan ahead.** After exercise, have high-carbohydrate foods handy so you don't have to think about what you're going to eat. It just makes it easier on you. If you have the time to train, you'll need to find the time for fueling as well.

6. **Eat enough!** The best time to replete your muscles of the glycogen they need for energy is after a workout. According to one study (Applegate, 1991), approximately three grams of carbohydrate per pound of body weight per day will saturate a trained muscle. That means 3 grams of carbohydrates x 150 lbs = 450 grams = 1800 carbohydrate calories. This formula works best for very active athletes with high caloric needs, not for sedentary people.

7. **Rest.** Don't forget that even the best of the best have to rest their body. Both your muscles and your mind need time to recharge. Don't be so hard on yourself. Taking a day off won't make you fat or make you lose fitness. However, you should expect hunger, as your muscles need carbohydrate to refuel. Also, you should expect some temporary weight gain, as on rest days the glycogen that is being made is holding water with it. Remember that carbohydrate holds water, whether in the body or out. Generally, the ratio of glycogen to water is one to three. Don't let the number on the scale get you down if it's higher than what you expect. It's normal!

Exercise Lingo

What about terms like "glycogen loading" and "hitting the wall?" If you've ever hung around an athlete, you may have heard these funny sounding phrases on occasion. Glycogen loading is referring to the process of first depleting your glycogen stores in the muscle by limiting carbohydrate intake while exercising strenuously to ensure stores are depleted. Then, the day before the an event, the athlete will supersaturate the muscle with glycogen from dietary carbohydrate to maximize the amount of glycogen (energy) that can be stored for fuel during the event. Some research shows that glycogen loading can even be done effectively without depleting muscle glycogen stores initially. That is, a normal diet can be consumed followed by eating a meal high in carbohydrates to then "load" your muscles with the glycogen. Glycogen loading also tends to give body-builders that "pumped" look right before a competition. Glycogen loading in addition to consuming some protein, appears to be an even more superior way to get the most "bang for your buck." When protein is added to the carbohydrate load, your body's glycogen-producing process speeds up faster than if you loaded it with carbohydrates alone.

"Hitting the wall" is a saying that is used to refer to a person who suddenly feels intense fatigue; as if there is a brick wall in front of them and they are trying to push through it.

Physiologically, a few things may be happening here. One is that they may be severely glycogen depleted. Another is that the exerciser may be working at an intensity that is too high, thus the build-up of lactic acid (a metabolic byproduct of anaerobic activity) is accumulating. Finally, a combination of these two could also be occurring.

It should be noted that there is a difference between muscular fatigue and blood fatigue. For example, if you are not getting

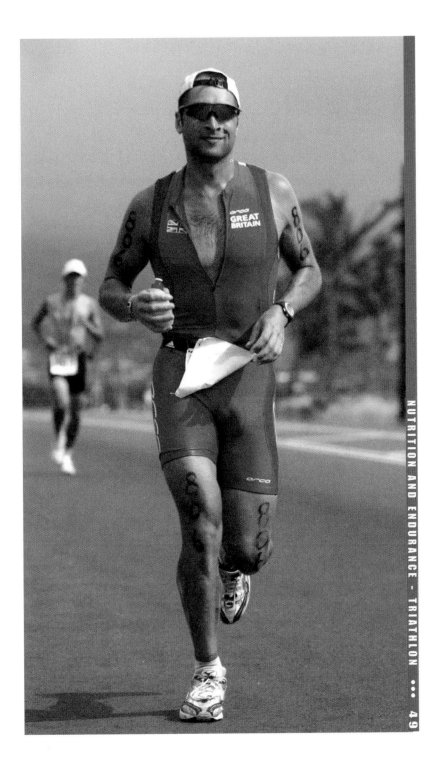

enough dietary carbohydrates, you may suffer from muscular fatigue. But if your diet lacks protein, iron and zinc, you may suffer from blood fatigue. A nutrition analysis with a registered dietitian could help you determine if this is a problem for you and how to correct it.

Did you know that after the age of 25, unless you strength train, you lose about a pound of muscle every year which will slow down your metabolism and lead to weight gain, even if you eat the same amount of calories as you get older?

Section I – Key ideas

1. There are 6 key nutrients for health: carbohydrate, protein, fat, vitamins, minerals and water.
2. Evaluate your diet. Keep a food record. Compare it to the Food Guide Pyramid or have a registered dietitian evaluate it for you.
3. F.I.T.T. stands for Frequency, Intensity, Time and Type. Use this acronym to help devise an exercise prescription for you to get started if you are not already training.

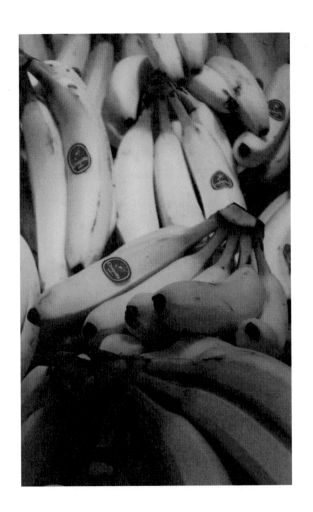

PART 2

Nutrition Basics

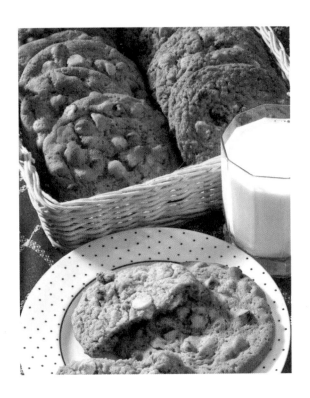

CHAPTER 4

Carbohydrates

The Good, The Bad, The Ugly

There is hardly a nutrition-minded client, student or patient of
mine that hasn't inquired about a low carbohydrate diet regimen.
Frequently, as I'm reviewing a food journal a client recorded for
me, he or she begins apologizing for the carbohydrates before I've
even had a chance to discuss their place in the diet.

When did carbohydrates become such an evil nutrient? There was a time when supplement companies couldn't keep enough maltodextrin (a form of pure carbohydrate) on the shelves. Today you may find an occasional ultra-endurance athlete looking for pure carbohydrates, but for the bodybuilder or recreational athlete carbohydrates are taboo. Stemming back to the original Atkins era, Body Opus, Protein Power, The Zone and the New Atkins Revolution, it appears that the media has proclaimed low carbohydrates as the in-vogue diet of the new millennium. And it's no wonder. With all the pseudo-scientific sounding terminology, tantalizing promises and clever marketing that surrounds the various high-protein, low carbohydrate plans, it's easy to be seduced and confused by it all.

Just how many carbohydrates should you be eating? The answer depends on who is asking the question. Low carbohydrate dieting refers to eating 50-100 grams of carbohydrates daily. Sometimes, dieters will later increase it to anywhere between 200-600 grams for a limited period of time depending upon total caloric intake. This is combined with high protein and moderate-to-high fat on the low carbohydrate days.

Do these types of diets work and who should be using them? Yes, they work but not how the people who sell them would like you to think. First, one cannot eat unlimited amounts of protein and fat and continue to lose fat. People think they can eat as much steak and eggs as they want everyday and look great. This might be true simply because most people can only choke down so much protein and fat per day. Additionally, high fat meals keep you full longer than low fat meals. Substantiated scientific research proves this type of eating (high, long-term saturated fat intake) is simply unhealthy and unnatural.

One group of athletes who might benefit from following this type of ketogenic diet (high protein-low carbohydrate diet) are competitive bodybuilders attempting to lower body fat stores temporarily in order to achieve contest ready physiques (5% body fat).

It is clear that carbohydrate needs vary, depending on the type of athlete. For endurance and ultra-endurance athletes, carbohydrates are undoubtedly the predominant fuel of choice, and thus a high carbohydrate ratio (50-65% of total calories) should be consumed in order to enhance and maximize athletic performance. For the strength trainer, carbohydrate needs may be as low as 40% of total calories, but not much lower. Conversely, the protein needs of the endurance athlete are less (1.0- 1.4 gms/kg/ day) – than that of the bodybuilder (1.4-1.8 gms/kg/day). See the section in Chapter 5 on protein for your specific protein needs.

The Glycemic Index

The next area of concern deals with the proper use of high and low glycemic index carbohydrates. The Glycemic Index (GI) is a numerical reference value of insulin response to carbohydrates. This index is influenced by the form in which the food is eaten (liquid, solid, cooked, uncooked), fiber content, protein/fat, processing and preparation. All of these variables will affect carbohydrate insulin response, which makes it difficult to control or determine the actual end-glucose response. Another negative aspect of this index is that the figures were determined by a single 3 oz. serving of a particular carbohydrate eaten by itself. In other words, mixed meals (the type of meals most people eat) and the portion will greatly influence the insulin response.

Are all carbohydrates equal? Yes, in the sense that all carbohydrates are made up of simple sugars. However, they come in different sizes such as monosaccharides (1 sugar) disaccharides (2 sugars linked), and polysaccharides (many sugars linked). The mono- and disaccharides make up the simple sugars while the polysaccharides make up complex carbohydrates. Total calories (quantity) and macronutrient ratio (quality) will always determine how these nutrients act in the body. Therefore, quantity and quality of carbohydrates are both important. However, eating low glycemic carbohydrates doesn't mean that you can eat as much as you want. Too many low GI carbohydrates can raise insulin levels the same as pure dextrose (GI of 100). It was once thought that if the quantity of carbohydrates were controlled, it really didn't matter if they were low- or high-glycemic. Recently research has shown that when carbohydrates are controlled, choosing low GI index carbohydrates produces a greater weight loss than high GI carbohydrates (Kritchevsky, 1980). Why? It appears that when carbohydrates and calories are controlled, the low GI carbohydrates produce less insulin, which produces an environment conducive to weight loss.

The areas of interest with respect to glycemic index include pre-workout athletic performance, post-workout recovery and calorie-controlled fat loss. Research continues to show that pre-workout consumption of low GI carbohydrates versus high GI carbohydrates may improve endurance and performance (Blom, 1987). The results indicate that a steady insulin response, versus an insulin spike, helps to provide a higher controlled availability of glucose for energy without providing too much glucose at one time (which would impair performance). Interestingly, there is also research showing no benefit from pre-workout low GI consumption (Costill, 1985). One reason for this (as with other research) is the difference in study protocols and variables. For instance, one study tests long-term endurance and another examines short-term endurance. In the first study, carbohydrates are consumed during the test, and in the latter, they are not. Clearly, more time is needed to perform further studies and compile a respectable amount of research for each protocol and variable. Factors that appeared in most of the research (both positive and negative studies) were the metabolic variables. Most of the test subjects that consumed low GI carbohydrates pre-workout had low insulin responses, higher amounts of available glucose and lower ratings of perceived exertion.

Table 3

Glycemic Index (GI) of common foods

Food	GI	Food	GI
Lentils	41	Sweet corn	78
Fettucine	46	Brown Rice	79
Barley	49	Popcorn	79
Vermicelli	50	Oatmeal Cookies	79
Apple	54	White Rice	83
Apple juice	58	Cheese Pizza	86
Spaghetti, white	59	Ice Cream	87
All-Bran cereal	60	Raisins	91
Peach	60	Macaroni and Cheese	92
Orange	63	Nutri-grain bar	94
Macaroni	64	Grapenuts cereal	96
Linguine	65	Cream of Wheat	100
Grapes	66	Bagel	103
Green peas	68	Watermelon	103
Grapefruit juice	69	Donut	108
Chocolate	70	Total cereal	109
Cheese tortellini	71	Pretzels	116
Orange juice	74	Rice Krispies cereal	117
Banana	77	Cornflakes cereal	119
Special K cereal	77	Baked Potato	121
Sweet Potato	77	Crispix cereal	124
Oat Bran	78	Instant Rice	128
Spaghetti, durum	78		

Studies concerning post-workout carbohydrate consumption sugest that high GI carbohydrates are more effective at replenishing glycogen stores. Muscle glycogen content has been shown to be greater within 24 hours of recovery with the high glycemic index diet versus low glycemic diet. This shows that a rapid increase in muscle glycogen during the first 24 hours of recovery may be achieved by consuming high GI index carbohydrates (Browns, 1989). Another example of this is the difference between sucrose (high GI) and fructose (low GI) when it comes to glycogen storage. Sucrose increases post-workout glycogen storage more than fructose, due to insulin response and the fact that fructose must first replenish liver glycogen before muscle glycogen. Another research topic has been the evaluation of the effects of high and low GI calorie-controlled fat loss. It appears that when calories are controlled, the GI index does affect the amount of fat lost. All other factors the same, it appears that a low GI meal can be better controlled and produces a low insulin response, which can foster increased fat loss. So the three cases when the GI of carbohydrates should be considered are: preworkout consumption, post-workout consumption and during periods of fat loss or competition dieting.

In summary, endurance athletes should consume a minimum of 50% carbohydrates for athletic performance while strength athletes may consider going as low as 40%. Pay attention to the GI index during pre-workout and post-workout meals. Remember that carbohydrates are not the evil macronutrient.

Table 4

Estimate of daily carbohydrate requirements (in grams) based on bodyweight and hours of training

Bodyweight (lbs)	Daily Training (hours)		
	2	3	4
110	300	400	500
132	400	500	600
154	500	600	700
176	600	700	800
198	700	800	900
220	800	900	1,000
242	900	1,000	1,100

Other points to remember:

▲ After you've determined your carbohydrate daily needs, try to spread intake throughout the day.

▲ 1 gram of carbohydrate = 4 calories

Pre-Competition

The amount of glycogen in the muscles before competition is the most important fuel determinant of performance. As you get closer to the actual date of the event, you should consider some important changes in your training diet such as carbohydrate loading.

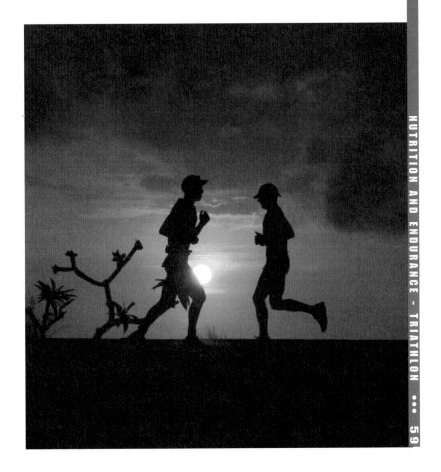

Muscle glycogen supercompensation: AKA: Carbohydrate loading!

While carbohydrate loading will not help you run faster, it can help keep you fueled and thereby maintain your pace longer before tiring out. Traditionally, the process of depleting your muscles of glycogen for up to four to five days and repleting them with a carbohydrate diet for three to four days worked well for some and poorly for others. The method has recently been revised and many believe the carbohydrate loading process (up to 10-15 g carbohydrate/kg per day) should last only about one or two days. Also, for some athletes, depletion may not even be necessary. Just loading up on the carbohydrates the day before may suffice.

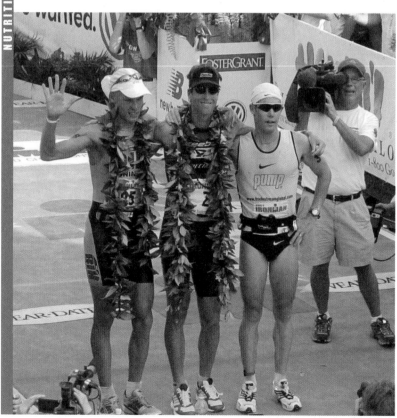

It's important that when you load on carbohydrate-rich food, they should also be low-fat (not necessarily NO-fat). For example, rather than choosing lasagna filled with cheese and beef, try spaghetti or linguine noodles with marinara sauce. Instead of doughnuts, choose bagels. Instead of French fries, try a baked potato with low-fat plain yogurt.

Remember that every gram of carbohydrate comes with three grams of water. With training being tapered and extra carbohydrates being consumed the week before, don't be surprised if you feel like you've gained some weight. But not to worry, this is a good thing. Carbohydrate loading actually helps hydrate your muscles better because of the extra water.

Carbohydrate loading is useful for events that are two continuous hours or longer. So if you enjoy 5 or 10K running events, a high-carbohydrate meal three to four hours before the event and proper hydration should be all you need. For example, if you typically consume 2500 calories per day with 60 percent of your calories coming from carbohydrate, you eat about 375 grams of carbohydrate a day. To get the fuel you need, focus on eating plenty of starchy carbohydrates such as bread, cereal, rice, pasta, beans, potatoes and fruit. (Fruit is not really starchy but it is an excellent source of carbs). Remember, only 1/2 cup of most cooked carbs like pasta and potato will give you 15 grams! Only 1/3 cup of cooked rice will provide 15 grams of carbs.

During Competition

If the event is less than 60 minutes, you will probably not need any carbohydrate to keep your muscles fueled with glycogen. If the event exceeds an hour, remember that you don't want to wait until you begin to feel fatigue because you can't maintain your pace. Around minute 30, start consuming 30 to 60 grams of carbohydrate for every hour you exercise. Most sports drinks (i.e. Gatorade, Exceed, PowerAde, Hydra Fuel, Allsport) supply 15-20 grams of carbohydrate per one-cup serving so you'll need double or triple that amount (up to 3 cups) per hour. Remember: 8 ounces equals 1 cup, so check the nutrition label. Also, try not to gulp it all down too quickly. You want to avoid any possible abdominal discomfort.

If the duration of your exercise exceeds 4 hours, then you'll need to aim for at least 60 grams of carbohydrate per hour in the latter stages of the event. Carbohydrate-rich foods such as a large banana (30 grams), 1/4 cup raisins (30 grams), energy-bars (20-50 grams), a packet of sports gel (25 grams) or other familiar and well-tolerated foods can help meet your needs. Energy gels should be taken with water to prevent them from ending up as a thick glob of syrup just sitting in your stomach! You'll need 8 oz. of plain water with every packet of energy gel you consume.

Post-Competition

Remember that when you eat carbohydrates, it converts into the glycogen your body stores in the muscles and liver for energy. To summarize the earlier section on GI, certain types of carbohydrate make a better choice than others for post-race carbohydrate refueling. The type of carbohydrates that will convert into glycogen the quickest are "simple" or "fast" carbohydrates. Recall that "high glycemic index" carbs refers to how quickly certain foods convert into sugar in the blood. The higher the glycemic index, the quicker the food converts into sugar in the blood-stream, the quicker it becomes available for conversion to glycogen. This is the time to load up on fruit, fruit juice, fruit shakes, yogurt, sports drinks, and even more refined carbohy-drates like wafers, crackers and pretzels. Second, consider that the enzymes that convert carbohydrates to glycogen are at their highest activity level if you eat no later than 60 - 75 minutes after the event.

So, don't wait around to eat. If you don't get in those carbs soon enough, you lose out on your body's peak opportunity to recover properly. For your body to completely recover from intense glyco-gen depletion (due to a race such as the Ironman) you should eat again several times throughout the day since it really takes up to a full day to replenish glycogen stores. Your target intake is 0.5 grams of carbs per pound of body weight every two hours for 6-8 hours. For example, 190lbs x 0.5 g. carbs/lb. = 95 g carbs = 380 carb calories. Two hours later, eat another 380 carb cals.

Example: fruit/soy protein shake made with fruit and/or fruit juice and fruited yogurt

Did you know that eating or drinking sugary foods just prior to training may actually impair per-formance in some individuals because the concentrated sugar can attract too much fluid in the stomach and intestines, which may be very uncomfortable to the athlete?

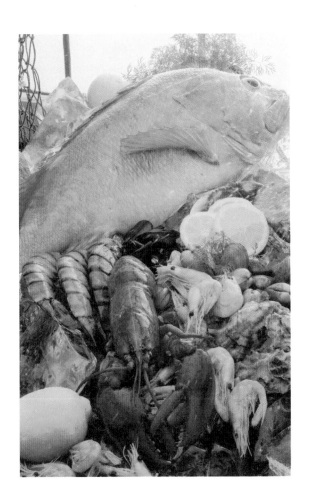

CHAPTER 5

Protein Power

Proteins have long been used by athletes following strenuous activity to help the body repair and rebuild muscle tissue. Individuals engaging in regular, strenuous exercise need more protein than those with a less active lifestyle.

Proteins are made of chains of amino acids that are sequenced together in various combinations. (Remember the beads on a string analogy from Chapter 1). The different combinations of sequenced amino acids will yield all different kinds of proteins, each with their own unique function.

Currently, the recommended dietary allowance (RDA) for protein for sedentary adults is 0.8 gm per kg of body weight per day (recall that 1 kg = 2.2 lbs). Athletes need 50-100% more protein than the adult RDA. Specifically, endurance athletes need between 1.2 - 1.4 gm protein/kg body weight during prolonged endurance exercise. Strength athletes may even need as much as 1.6 - 1.7 gm/kg body weight during maintenance phases of training and up to 2.0 gm per kg if they are in the muscle building phase of training. Consider that 1 oz of any meat food, such as fish poultry, beef, veal, ham, or pork contains 7 grams of protein. Also, remember that grain foods have up to 3 grams per 1/2 cup.

That means, according to the American Dietetic Association (ADA), these recommended protein intakes can generally be met through diet alone. It isn't necessary to use protein or amino acid supplements if carbohydrate intake is adequate to maintain body weight. When muscle glycogen (stored carbohydrate) stores are low due to prolonged exercise or a low carbohydrate diet, protein may contribute as much as 10% of the energy needed for exercise. However, when muscle glycogen stores are high, the contribution of protein for energy is less than 5%. Athletes will also use more protein for fuel when they don't eat enough calories. Consuming a high carbohydrate diet during repeated days of heavy training helps to maintain muscle glycogen stores and reduces the use of protein as fuel. This spares protein so that it can be used for other important functions such as repairing and rebuilding muscle tissue and keeping the immune system fully functioning.

Table 5

Endurance athlete

175 pounds = 79.5 kg *(2.2 lbs = 1 kg)*

Protein needs = 1.2-1.4 grams per kg = 95-112 grams per day

Sample Diet:	Food	Protein in grams
Breakfast:	1 cup skim milk	8
	1 small banana	0
	2 egg omelet	14
Snack:	1 apple	0
	1 oz string cheese	7
Lunch:	sandwich consisting of:	
	2 slices whole-wheat bread	6
	3 oz turkey	21
	1 slice of cheese	7
	lettuce, tomato	0
	1/2 cup fruited yogurt	4
Snack:	1 oz nuts	5
	6 crackers	3
Dinner:	4 oz chicken	28
	1 1/2 cups cooked pasta	9
	salad	0
	Total Protein = 112 grams	

Some athletes, who for various reasons don't consume adequate calories or protein daily, may purchase protein supplements. But once inside the health food store, it is easy to get overwhelmed by the different types of protein supplements available. How does one filter through the flood of products that all claim to be the "right one for you?"

The next section will briefly examine four types of protein supplements: whey protein, branched-chain amino acids, glutamine and soy (vegetable protein).

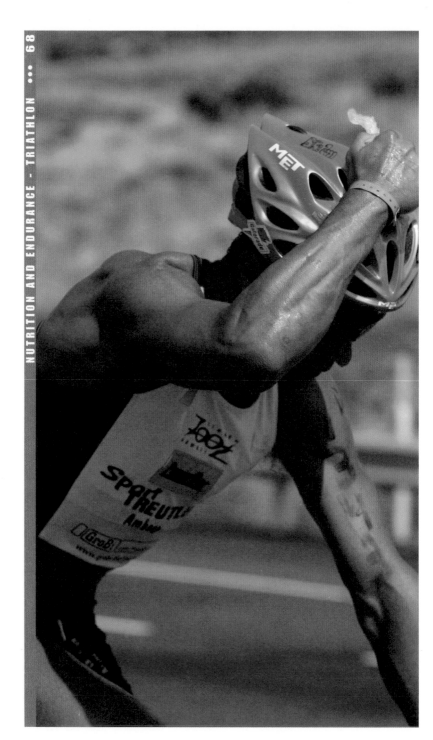

1. **Whey protein** – One of the best-known and best selling proteins is whey protein. It is a milk-based protein that is particularly abundant in alpha-lactalbumin, commonly referred to as a "fraction" of whey protein. Alpha-lactalbumin is also found in human milk and is an extremely nutritious, low allergenic protein. A good quality whey-protein product would supply 15% to 20% of alpha-lactalbumin. The main protein source in a high-quality whey product should be whey protein isolate. Whey protein isolate is the "cleanest," lowest fat, lowest cholesterol and lowest sodium whey protein available. Another test of quality lies in how it is processed. There are various processing and production techniques, however, the process that combines both "ion-exchange" and "cold micro-filtration" appear to produce the highest quality product. Typically, the label of the supplement will indicate how it's been processed. Additionally, because whey proteins naturally provide about 23% of their total amino acid content as branched-chain amino acids (BCAAs are described later), supplementing on more BCAAs may be unnecessary. Some whey protein supplements also contain added glutamine (also described later), and other types of nutrients such as taurine, phenylalanine, arginine, vitamin B6 and magnesium.

2. **Branched Chain Amino Acids** - BCAAs consist of only three amino acids. They are leucine, isoleucine and valine. They have been touted to improved exercise performance by increasing stamina and improving mental concentration. BCAAs are not readily broken down by the liver, rather are taken up into the brain. Another amino acid, tryptophan, is also taken up into the brain and is known to be the precursor to a brain chemical, serotonin, which is believed to be partly responsible for fatigue in prolonged aerobic endurance exercise. BCAAs are theorized to block the entry of free tryptophan into the brain, decreasing the formation of the neurotransmitter serotonin. Out of eight studies conducted on BCAAs and exercise performance,

one concluded that an increased supply of BCAAs may have a sparing effect on muscle glycogen degradation during exercise. Another study proposed that an intake of BCAAs during exercise may prevent or decrease the net rate of protein breakdown caused by heavy exercise. Carbohydrate supplementation can also prove effective in this regard since carbohydrate is the primary fuel for prolonged aerobic endurance athletes, and such athletes normally carbohydrate-load before competition and consume carbohydrate beverages during the event.

3. **Glutamine** – The most abundant amino acid in skeletal muscle and is a fuel source for many types of cells. "Feeding" the cells of the gut is one of glutamine's most well-known functions. Apparently, body stores of glutamine decrease during exercise. In a study that looked at triathletes after a half-Ironman race, glutamine levels and the immune system related cells were suppressed (Rohde, 1996). Glutamine has been referred to as "anticatabolic," in that it assists in the prevention of muscle breakdown. It has also been marketed to keep the immune system strong and prevent infection during heavy exercise training. In another study with 151 middle-distance, marathon and ultramarathon runners and elite rowers, the authors concluded that glutamine supplementation after prolonged exercise might restore glutamine to physiological levels, thus making glutamine more available to immune cells (Castel, 1997).

4. **Soy Protein** – Soy protein is the only known vegetable protein that contains all the essential amino acids. Generally, only animal protein contains all the essential amino acids. If one does not consume any animal foods or animal products, vegetable foods with some of those amino acids (example: rice) would be combined with other vegetable foods (example: beans) with other amino acids in order to get all the essential amino acids in the diet. Soy has received much attention on its

controversial positive and negative health effects as it relates to cardiovascular disease, cancer, menopause and osteoporosis. However, although soy is a perfectly acceptable protein alternative to whey, it is generally not considered the protein of choice for muscle growth and strength building.

Table 6
Daily protein requirement in grams

Bodyweight		Sports/Training Category		
(lbs)	(kgs)	Strength*	Speed**	Endurance***
154	70	140	119	98
176	80	160	136	112
198	90	180	153	126
220	100	200	170	140

Recall: 1 gram of protein = 4 calories.
     1 kg = 2.2 lbs
*Strength = 2.0 gm/kg/day
**Speed = 1.7 gm/kg/day   represent upper limits
***Endurance = 1.4 gm/kg/day

Points to Remember:

▲ Despite what the ads imply, it is not just protein intake that controls muscle growth. It is the demand for growth caused by the trauma of intense exercise. No one ever grew an ounce of muscle from simply gulping protein. Muscles grow from pushing pounds.

▲ Individual protein intake must match the training program. See table for protein requirements in grams.

▲ Plant carbohydrates don't have to be eaten together to reap complete protein benefits.

▲ Don't avoid protein in your recovery diet. Aim for 1 gram of protein for every 3 grams of carbohydrates. Besides the carbohydrates being critical to replace after a workout, the protein is also important. This is not only for nutrient balance, but because following your workout the body is most optimally ready for protein intake to repair and rebuild damaged muscle tissue. A protein shake with fresh and frozen fruit (i.e. bananas and frozen mixed berries), milk or yogurt is a very good choice.

Did you know that eating excessive amounts of protein does not automatically convert into muscle? Rather, if you eat more protein than your body requires, it will convert into fat or be excreted.

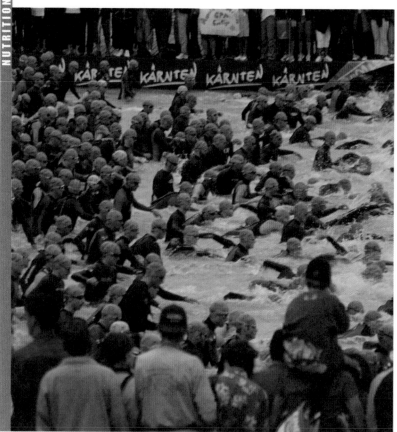

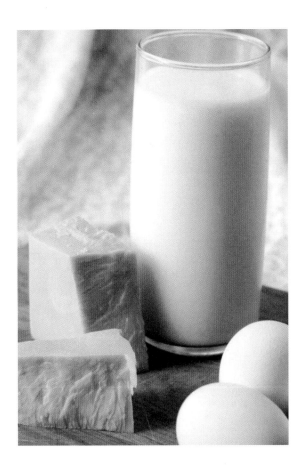

CHAPTER 6
Fat Matters

Not too long ago, food manufacturers began coming out with the "new and improved" fat-free or low-fat versions of practically all foods. This is in response to the rising government statistics indicating that Americans are simply getting too fat. After the first wave of the low carbohydrate, high protein diet craze in the late 70s, various health organizations began making nutrition recommendations to the mass public to lower dietary fat intake. Even the Food Guide Pyramid, which replaced the Four Food Groups in the mid 90s, teaches to limit fats and illustrates this by depicting it at the top of the pyramid. One would think that if you eat less fat, rates of obesity should decline, but they haven't. In fact, in October 1999, the Centers for Disease Control (CDC) and Prevention in Atlanta officially declared obesity an epidemic. This was in response to mounting evidence including a study published in the Journal of the American Medical Association. In essence, there are currently more people who are overweight than there are people who are normal weight.

Clearly the reasons for this must be multifaceted. One purported theory is that while we cut out some of our dietary fat, we replaced it with too much refined sugar. Therefore, total caloric intake remained the same if not higher. Also, there was not enough emphasis on the types of fats that should be eliminated; the message mainly being to just reduce all types of fats. The reason is that all fats and oils are created equally when it comes to its fat and calorie content. One gram of any oil or fat is equal to nine calories - saturated or not. Cholesterol free or not. And don't be fooled into thinking that "light" or "extra virgin" olive oils have less fat or fewer calories that other oils. The label simply reflects the oil's taste, color and aroma.

The way fats differ is that they are either saturated or unsaturated. If it's unsaturated, it's then classified as either monounsaturated or polyunsaturated. The rule of thumb is that all animal fats are saturated. This includes any type of meat, poultry, fish, milkfat, or butter... if it came from an animal and it has fat, it's saturated. Does this mean that ALL plant fats are unsaturated (monounsaturated or polyunsaturated)? No, but most plant fats are unsaturated. The exception to the rule is that coconut oil and palm oil, also referred to as the "tropical oils" are highly saturated. Saturation and cholesterol-containing fats are two different matters.

In this case, all animal fats contain cholesterol and all plant fats do not. So, for example, although coconut oil is highly saturated, it does not have cholesterol, because it is a plant based fat.

While it is true that too much of ANY fat can potentially add a lot of extra calories that'll make it tough to shed the pounds, saturated fat (animal fat, coconut oil and palm oil) is much more harmful to your health. This is due to its ability to raise levels of bad cholesterol, thus increasing your risk for heart disease. Conversely, monounsaturated fat, such as olive or canola (a modified rapeseed oil developed by the Canola Council of Canada, hence the name canola oil) does have a better effect on blood cholesterol levels than oils that are predominantly polyunsaturated fat, such as corn, safflower and soybean oils.

Getting Your Omega-3s - A Matter of Fat

One type of fat that has been receiving a lot more attention both in scientific studies and in clinical circles is omega-3 fat. Popular versions of omega-3 fats are DHA and EPA. There is a considerable amount of evidence that omega-3 fats have many positive health properties. We now know omega-3 fats are crucial for normal brain development, lower blood pressure and triglyceride levels. It also acts as an anti-inflammatory and blood thinner. In fact, omega-3s appear to be so effective at thinning the blood that if you are on another type of blood thinning medicine or vitamin (such as vitamin E), the synergistic effect of the two may be too intense.

Excellent sources of DHA include breastmilk, salmon, flax seed oil, fish oil supplements, macademia nuts, canola oil, soybeans, and wheatgerm. (Don't confuse DHA, a fatty acid, with DHEA, a hormone that has recently been put in the form of a supplement). It is not very encouraging to know that the current intake in the United States is only about one-tenth of the optimal omega-3 recommendation. And what is the recommendation? Only 1-1.5 grams a day! Not a large amount at all!

Trans Fats – The Phantom Fats?

Ever hear of cis and trans fatty acids? A process known as partial or complete hydrogenation takes a naturally occurring cis-fatty acid and converts it to a trans-fatty acid.

If manufacturers want the advantage of a fat that contains no cholesterol and want it to be solid at room temperature they use hydrogenation. Hydrogenation is a chemical process that alters the structure of fat to an oil. For example, corn oil is normally not saturated and is liquid at room temperature. After hydrogenation it becomes margarine, which is saturated and solid at room temperature. In the process of hydrogenating a product, the altered chemical make up of the fat produces an unusual fat called trans fat.

Trans fats and saturated fats have been correlated with an increased risk for heart disease. Of course, when total fat in the diet is reduced (margarine and butter have the same number of fat calories per gram – 9 calories per gram), this also helps limit total calories, saturated fats and trans fats. If you just love your peanut butter or margarine, new non-hydrogenated products are available in most major grocery stores around the country that contain no trans fats.

The Cholesterol Question

Most people have heard about how cholesterol is this nasty stuff in fat-laden foods that gives people heart attacks..right? Sort of. Cholesterol is a type of a fat, but it doesn't contain calories as dietary fats like the regular fat in food. And because it's a fatty substance whose function is only needed in animals and humans, you won't find it in plant foods even if the plant source contains saturated fats.

Although it is a well-established fact that high blood cholesterol levels are a primary risk factor in heart disease, cholesterol is a vitally important body substance. It's as crucial as biologically similar structures such as estrogen, testosterone, and adrenal hormones like cortisol as it is the starting material for the making of these compounds. In fact, as you read this paragraph, your liver is making cholesterol at the rate of about 5×10^{16} (50,000,000,000,000,000) molecules per second (800 to 1500 milligrams per day). So, despite the popular notion that cholesterol is an absolute evil, it is really not. As you can see, the liver contributes much more cholesterol than the diet.

This Dr. Jekyll and Mr. Hyde nutrient has two faces because it also has the ability to have harmful effects in the body when it forms deposits on the inner walls of the arteries. Accumulations of soft fatty streaks are what eventually leads to deposits of plaque, which leads to atherosclerosis; a type of artery disease that causes strokes and heart disease. With time these plaques just keep building up, making it more and more difficult for the oxygen-carrying blood to reach all the oxygen-craving cells of your body. When those plaques have built up to the point the blood simply can't get through, WHAM! You've just had a heart attack!

No one is truly free of the fatty streaks that may one day become the fibrous plaques of atherosclerosis. For most, the question is not whether you have them, but how far advanced they are and what you can do to retard or reverse their progression.

Does a diet high in cholesterol cause atherosclerosis? Research is showing more and more that cholesterol doesn't seem to be the instigator as much as dietary triglycerides (that means fat from foods). However, this is not your "thumbs up" to go off that low-cholesterol eating plan that's now become your way of life. It just means that cholesterol is the lesser of two evils.

What about all that "good" and "bad" cholesterol stuff? "Good" and "bad" cholesterol are just components of total cholesterol. If you add up the "good" and "bad" cholesterol number you get from your doctor's lab report its sum should represent your total cholesterol. You know, the one that your doctor said you should keep under 200 mg/dl.

In terms of function, think of these creatures as little "taxicabs". That is, they serve to transport cholesterol to and from the liver. If the "taxicab" is taking cholesterol from the body to the liver, it's called a high-density lipoprotein (HDL) or "good" cholesterol. In the liver that cholesterol is going to get recycled for some other good use rather than becoming the promoter of fatty streaks to your arteries. Conversely, if the "taxicab" is taking cholesterol from the liver to the arteries of the body, it is referred to as low-density lipoprotein (LDL) or the "bad" cholesterol. So, you don't find these "taxicabs" in the foods that you eat. "Good" cholesterol is not a type of cholesterol found in foods, but refers to the way the blood transports cholesterol. Here's a very simple list of numbers to remember when it comes to cholesterol and heart health.

Table 7

Blood Values
Total Cholesterol - < 200 mg/dL = desirable
HDL Cholesterol - > 35 mg/dL = desirable
LDL Cholesterol - < 130 mg/dL = desirable
Triglycerides - < 150 mg/dL = desirable
Total Cholesterol/HDL Ratio – 4.5 or lower = desirable

Dietary Values
Cholesterol - < 300 mg/day = desirable
Triglycerides (Fat) – not > 30 % of total cals = desirable

Bottom Line:

1. Focus on reducing unhealthy fats (saturated and trans fats) in the diet by reducing the amount of animal fat and processed products such as regular peanut butter and regular margarine.
2. Look for labels that specifically say "non-hydrogenated" or "no trans fats."
3. Eat more of the monounsaturated fats such as olive and canola oil.
4. Consider taking an omega-3 supplement for added heart health protection. Check with a registered dietitian (R.D.) for specific recommendations. To find a registered dietitian in your area, simply visit www.eatright.org and type in your zip code.

Fat: 20-30% of total calories should supply fat, preferably unsaturated!

Recall: 1 gram of fat = 9 calories: concentrated energy!

The following table is to recommend the amount of fat to consume in grams based on the total number of calories in one's diet. For example: If you eat 2800 calories, 25% of calories coming from fat equals 77 grams of fat.

Table 8

	20% from fat	25% from fat	30% from fat
2000 calories	44 grams	56	66
2400	54	67	80
2800	62	77	93
3200	71	89	107
3600	80	100	120
4000	89	111	133

Rule of thumb:

▲ All animal fats are saturated

▲ Most plant fats are unsaturated

   exception: "tropical" oils – coconut oil, palm oil

Points to Remember:

▲ Avoid high fat foods before, during and after any event. Fats slow down the digestion of foods and do not contribute to glycogen rebuilding.

▲ Minimize saturated fats.

▲ Use extra virgin olive oil and canola oil whenever possible.

▲ Use flax seeds for linolenic acid (omega-3 fatty acid).

▲ Good sources of omega-3 fats: Fish such as salmon, trout, mackerel.

▲ Keep fat intake under 25% of total calories.

Table 9

Instead of these HIGH-FAT foods choose the LOW–FAT option:

HIGH	LOW
Whole milk	Skim or 1% milk
Sour cream	Non-fat yogurt
Cream soups	Vegetable soup
Fried chicken	Baked or grilled chicken
Eggs, bacon and sausages	Eggs and whole-wheat toast
Grits with butter	Oatmeal with honey
Apple pie	Fresh apples
Potato chips	Fresh sweet potato
Recipe with 1 cup oil	1/2 cup oil and 1/2 cup apple sauce
Creamy salad dressings	Raspberry vinaigrette dressing
Cheesecake	Oatmeal raisin cookie
Sausage pizza	Veggie pizza
Meat lasagna	Veggie lasagna

Did you know that 1 cup of whole milk contains over 50% fat compared to 1 cup of skim milk which is less than 5% fat?

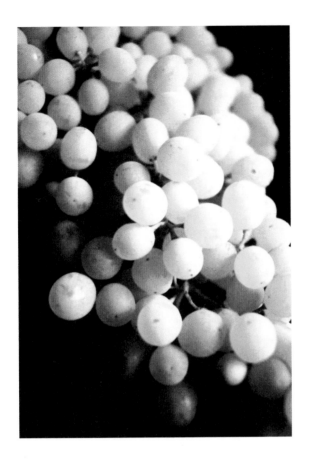

CHAPTER 7

Fluid Facts

The human body is roughly two-thirds water. Maintaining proper hydration is one of the most important nutritional practices for optimizing exercise performance year-round. It is especially important in the hot and humid summer months!

Fluids are needed for multiple functions in your body: regulating body temperature (increases in body temperature lead to decreased performance), transportation of metabolic substrates (oxygen, glucose) & wastes (carbon dioxide, lactic acid) in the blood, maintaining cardiac output (cardiac output refers to the heart's ability to pump blood through your body) and muscular and brain function (muscles and brain primarily consist of water – they do not function well without it).

In order to maintain tight fluid balance, hydration levels have to be at + 0.2% of total body weight. The regulation of one's fluid status is controlled by balancing fluid input (fluid that is ingested daily) with fluid output (the volume of fluid that is lost in the urine, feces, sweat, and respiration). In general, if your fluid intake is less than your fluid output, certain hormones are released that allow the kidney to increase its water and sodium retention while provoking an increase in thirst. Conversely, when fluid input is greater than fluid output, the kidneys restore water balance by excreting excess fluid.

One of the challenges athletes commonly face is finding and meeting that fluidbalance. Thirst sensors in the brain are not sensitive, thus the athlete may not always detect or feel the thirst sensation. In general, most runners drink less than about 500 ml of fluid per hour, yet sweat rates of marathon runners often average 1,000-1,500 ml per hour. This puts them at a dehydration rate of 500-1000 ml per hour (Noakes, 1993).

For most non-athletes, fluid needs can be met by ingesting about 2 L (64 oz) per day. This amount may be a gross underestimation of what an athlete needs on a training day, which is closer to 6 L.

Electrolyte Considerations

Although your body is about two-thirds water, fluid is not the only thing that is lost in the urine and sweat. Dissolved in the body fluids (like sweat and urine) are electrolytes; minerals that carry an electrical charge. Their main purpose is to promote the transmission of messages across nerve cells and to regulate water balance on either side of the cells. This is how your body is able to conduct functions such as contracting muscles, maintaining a heartbeat or giving us that bloated feeling of holding water when we've consumed too much salt. The most popular electrolytes are sodium, potassium and chloride. During exercise, some sodium and potassium are lost through sweat. According to the American College of Sports Medicine's (ACSM – the official leader and "gold standard" in the sports nutrition industry) position statement on exercise and fluid replacement, if you are a casual exerciser or exercising less than one hour, you probably don't need to supplement with electrolytes. In this case, water is the best fluid replacement for you and drinking sports drinks will not help you exercise more safely or effectively. On the other hand, competitive athletes may benefit from potassium-rich sports drinks, especially if they've been on the go for at least one hour.

The ACSM also recommends that individuals consume about 500 ml (about 17 oz) of fluid about 2 hours before exercise to promote adequate hydration and allow time for excretion of excess ingested water. To minimize the risk of overheating, which can impair exercise performance (particularly the development of muscle cramps), it is recommended that fluid replacement equals fluid loss.

Potassium is not conserved by the body as well as sodium. Diuretics induce water loss and flush electrolytes out of the body via the urine. Therefore, anyone taking diuretics will want to be especially careful and under a physician's supervision. Electrolyte imbalances, especially potassium, caused by diuretic abuse, can lead to severe consequences including heart rhythm abnormalities. Certainly sodium and potassium in foods can be an excellent source of ensuring electrolytes in the diet. The following is a list of some common foods and their respective potassium and sodium contents in milligrams.

Table 10
Sodium and potassium amounts in various foods

Food	Potassium (mg)	Sodium (mg)
Avocado (1/2 medium)	530	53
Banana (medium)	451	1
Blackstrap molasses (1 tbsp)	498	11
Chicken breast (1/2)	240	70
Cooked mushrooms (1/2 cup)	278	2
Figs (10)	1331	21
Kidney beans (1 cup cooked)	713	4
Mozzarella cheese (1 oz.)	19	106
Nonfat milk (1 cup)	406	126
Orange juice (1 cup)	473	2
Salmon (3 oz)	327	52
Sunflower seeds (1oz.)	139	1
Sweet potato (1/2 cup)	278	2
Whole wheat bread (1 slice)	71	148

Ultimately, the goal of fluid and electrolyte balance is to promote safety by minimizing hyperthermia (elevated internal body temperature) and to maximize exercise performance. This translates into making sure that the athlete consumes the appropriate amount of fluid and electrolytes to compensate for the losses before, during and after exercise.

Remember that carbohydrates are a great source of water. For each gram of glycogen stored, the body also has to store 2.7 grams of water.

Pre-Competition: Pre-hydrate. Drink extra water for two days before the event. Then, between four hours and one hour before competition, drink an 8 oz glass every 10-15 min. Drink another two glasses between 30 min and 20 min before the start. Empty the bladder. Drink nothing during the 20 minutes before you start, because your stomach requires that much time to nearly empty. You don't want to cramp with water in the stomach.

Don't wait for the big event to pre-hydrate. Practice it during training. Training and competing without water-loading can cause possible permanent damage to your body because body temps can rise to over 105°F.

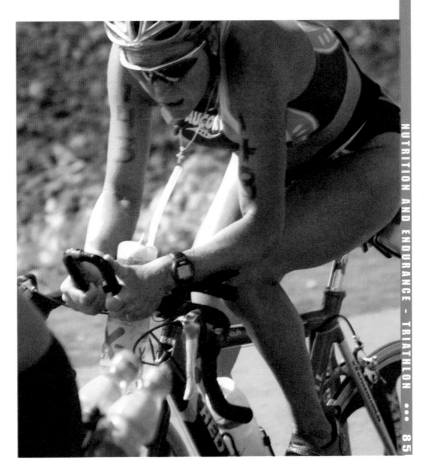

During competition - even if you are water-loaded before an event, you should take all the plain water you can during any long event. That means aim for 4-6 ounces every 15 – 20 mins. In running races beyond 1500 meters, aim to grab two cups at each aid station. In triathlons, put three water bottles on your bike.

Is it better to drink cold water versus room temperature water? The data is hazy. But, you should sip – don't gulp. This helps to avoid swallowing air.

Type of Beverage

1. Under one hour of exercise, plain water is best. Sugary drinks will prevent optimal absorption.

2. If high-sugar drinks are ingested, be careful of reactive hypoglycemia; a situation where too much sugar ingested will elicit a quick and sharp insulin response, thereby drastically lowering blood sugars and causing sudden fatigue.

3. For especially long events, sports drinks that are less than 10% sugar are preferred, i.e. Hydra Fuel by Twinlab which contains 7% sugar. Water plus carbohydrate is the best combination to prevent "hitting the wall" – a term that means you've suddenly run out of energy.

Post-Competition: Rehydrate! The best time to start rehydrating is directly after activity. First, drink plain water. Avoid juices – this will inhibit rehydration because of the high sugar content and may even promote cramps because it may add to stomach acidity. The basic rule of rehydration is to drink 2 to 3 cups (16 fl oz.) of fluid per every pound lost through sweat. Weigh yourself before and after activity to determine the amount you should drink following activity.

Continue drinking fluids until your urine is clear. This is a good indication that your body is hydrated again. If your urine is dark yellow, you definitely need to increase fluid intake. The best fluids are water and sports drinks. Sports drinks are ideal following longer duration activities since they contain carbohydrates and electrolytes as well as fluid. Water is also necessary to rehydrate yourself.

Don't stop moving after the event. You need the blood to continue circulating to prevent pooling of the blood around joints and to give oxygen to fatigued muscles.

You must rehydrate completely to recover.

 Did you know that many people overeat food when they are really just very thirsty?

1. *Eat frequently. Try to eat small meals frequently throughout the day (not more than 4 hours without eating). This will help prevent overeating at meals. Avoid both "picking" at food or eating too much in one sitting. This will keep you feeling full all day. It will also keep your blood sugars more stable, thereby avoiding hunger pangs that cause cravings, irritability, low energy and headaches.*

2. *Snack healthfully. Snacks can make or break the diet. Choose fresh fruit and vegetables with low or nonfat dairy products for a healthy carbohydrate and protein balance. Examples of good snacks are part-skim mozzarella cheese strings or plain, nonfat yogurt with raw vegetables, flavored non or low-fat yogurt topped with slivered almonds and seeds, fresh fruit and non or low-fat cottage cheese, whole-wheat crackers with natural peanut butter, pita bread with hummus, or energy bars that are not very high in carbohydrates or protein, but rather have a balance of carbohydrate, protein and fats.*

3 *Pre-Exercise Sports Meal. Choose slow or fibrous carbohydrates the night before you exercise or 3-4 hours before you train (if you do so in the afternoon) for sustained, steady fuel. Examples of "slow" or complex carbohydrates are wholewheat pasta, brown rice and sweet potatoes before you train. Try to keep this meal low fat to avoid feeling sluggish while training.*

4. *Post-Exercise Meal. 15 minutes to 1 hour after training, consume fast or simple carbohydrates to replenish the glycogen (stored carbs in the muscle and liver) you used during your workout. Protein is also important, not only for nutrient balance, but because after a workout your body is most optimally ready for protein intake to repair and rebuild muscle tissue. A protein shake with fresh and frozen fruit (i.e. bananas and frozen mixed berries) is a very good choice.*

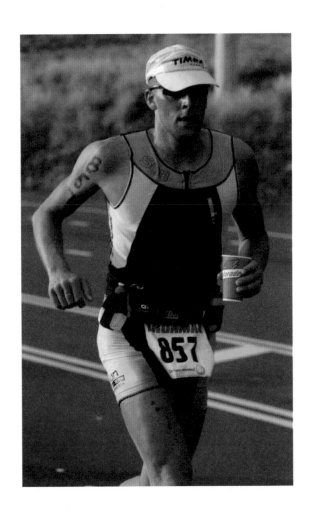

PART 3

Get Supplement Savvy

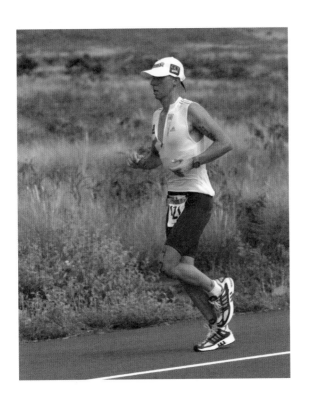

CHAPTER 8

The Ergogenic
Edge

The vitamin and mineral supplement industry is under-regulated and the regulations that do exist haven't been uniformly enforced. The U.S. Food and Drug Administration (FDA) regards supplements as foods, not drugs, which means the agency sets few rules for how the pills must be formulated or manufactured. A vitamin producer is not required to show that a tablet or capsule will break up into small pieces, as it should after it's swallowed, or dissolve in fluids so that the active ingredients can be absorbed by the body.

The law does require a supplement to contain the actual amount that's claimed on the label, but the government doesn't check systematically. A vitamin or mineral product that doesn't contain what it claims or that passes through the body intact is a waste of money. The stakes are higher when someone is taking supplements to prevent disease. For instance, taking calcium to prevent osteoporosis or folic acid to prevent birth defects.

A few years ago the United States Pharmacopeia (USP) began to develop voluntary standards to help assure the quality of vitamin and mineral products. The official USP standards now set forth procedures and criteria for measuring the potency of supplements (how much of the nutrients they contain) and how tablets and capsules break down physically (which is the first step that makes it possible for the body to use them). In January of 1998, the USP implemented standards for how rapidly certain products should dissolve, a measure thought to reflect their ability to get into the bloodstream.

A few major supplement manufacturers have announced that their products will conform to USP standards, allowing them to sport the "USP" logo. However, several other supplement companies have challenged the appropriateness of the USP's testing methods. It remains to be seen if many manufacturers will adopt those standards, and whether the USP logo on a vitamin bottle will be a useful guide in selecting products. In the meantime, consumers are left with little way to tell whether a nutritional supplement truly meets any of its claims.

Although there are a number of helpful supplements on the market, it is important to note that they do not and should not take the place of a healthy diet (hence the name supplement).

Additionally, several factors could influence your possible need for supplements, such as heredity, age and gender as well as lifestyle factors like smoking or alcohol consumption. Always consult your healthcare provider before beginning any type of supplement regimen, as the information in this chapter is not intended to replace medical advice.

Sometimes in the quest for achieving maximal performance, athletes will often rely on products to give them that extra "boost" or edge. These types of products are called ergogenic aids. If you break down the word ergogenic, "erg" refers to a unit of work while "genic" refers to the generation or production of. Put it together and these "work-producing" products may have the properties needed to enhance physical performance. Or do they?

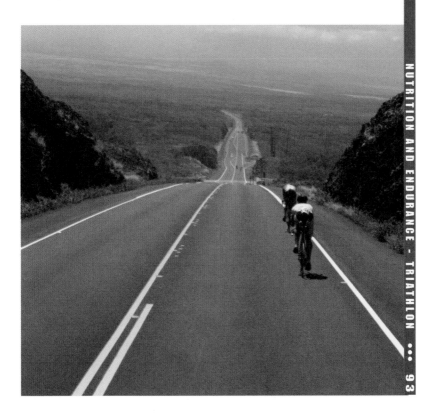

The demand for quality research on ergogenics is on the rise as it approaches a billion-dollar industry through clever advertising and sometimes false claims. One method involves the use of statistics from poorly-controlled studies in obscure, non-peer reviewed literature. Many companies throw in testimonials or suggestive marketing terms like "herbal, natural and mega." However, terms like these don't mean that they are harmless or nonaddictive. Many drugs are naturally occurring plant substances, but hopefully you wouldn't start a cocaine or nicotine habit just because someone told you it was "natural."

The rapid popularity of ergogenic aids is forcing more and more dollars to be spent on well conducted studies that are now being published in professional scientific journals. To help you sort through the more popular ones, here's a list of ergogenic aids available on the market today.

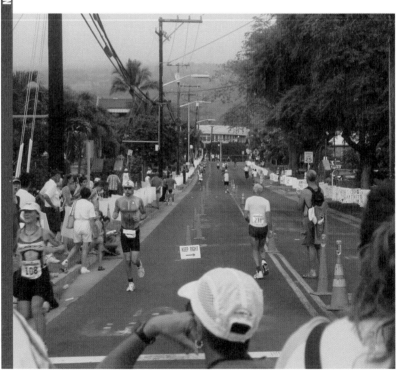

1. Amino acids: See Chapter 5 on Protein.

2. Antioxidants: Overall, antioxidant supplementation for the non-athlete seems to have beneficial effects, especially in terms of disease prevention. However, for the athlete, antioxidants don't appear to have ergogenic effects. Why? Athletes exercise. When you exercise you breathe in more oxygen. When you consume more oxygen, there is an increased number of dangerous unpaired electrons floating around that may result in more free radical damage to the body. The athlete compensates for this phenomenon by having a naturally enhanced antioxidant system. This is not seen in the beginner exerciser who doesn't have this developed antioxidant system. *See page 118 for a more detailed breakdown of the antioxidants and what they can do for you.*

3. Branched Chain Amino Acids (BCAAs) (leucine, isoleucine and valine): BCAAs are theorized to block the entry of free tryptophan (an essential amino acid) into the brain. This decreases the formation of the neurotransmitter, serotonin, which is believed to be partly responsible for fatigue in prolonged aerobic endurance exercise. Carbohydrate is the primary fuel for prolonged aerobic endurance athletes, and such athletes normally carbohydrate-load before competition and consume carbohydrate beverages during the event. According to most research studies, adding BCAAs to the solution does not appear to provide any additional benefits or adverse effects on prolonged aerobic endurance performance. Some limited data suggest that chronic BCAA supplementation may benefit performance. One theory is that BCAA supplementation may decrease muscle protein breakdown

during training, but carbohydrate supplementation might also be effective in this regard. Overall, there are no definitive studies that show that any single or combination of amino acids have an effect on muscle building.

4. Caffeine: It is not uncommon to see the professional as well as the recreational athlete ingest caffeine to aid exercise performance. Although the physiological effects may not have been understood until more recently, the stimulatory effects of caffeine have been known for thousands of years. It is important to note that caffeine is metabolized by the liver into three other compounds known as theobromine, theophylline, and paraxanthine (collectively referred to as methylxanthines). It is not entirely clear which one or group of these substances is actually responsible for the "coveted caffeine high" that is felt after, say, a cup of coffee. Although coffee is known for containing significant amounts of caffeine, the two should not be equated since coffee also contains hundreds of different chemicals. Caffeine is theorized to have several mechanisms for its ergogenic effect during exercise. One theory suggests that caffeine affects certain areas of the central nervous system that are responsible for the neural stimulation of muscle contraction and decreasing the perception of fatigue. Another theory related to the central nervous system suggests that caffeine interferes with adenosine, a chemical that plays a role in the brain by inducing sleep. Since caffeine has a similar molecular structure to adenosine, it can fit into adenosine receptors in the brain, which in turn does not cause the sedating effect of adenosine. In this sense, caffeine does not truly act as a stimulant, but rather a blocker of the calming effects of adenosine. Because it triggers the central nervous system, caffeine increases the release of adrenalin thus increasing the use of body fat as fuel and sparing muscle glycogen (stored carbohydrate). On the down side, caffeine is a diuretic. This means it can cause the body to lose precious fluids, especially through the urine. This can lead to dehydration which can seriously impair athletic performance. Additionally, if you drink coffee regularly, its ergogenic abilities are diminished. It probably won't give you that boost because your body is used to it. In order to be effective as an ergogenic aid, you have to take the caffeine at the right time since the fat-burning response to caffeine doesn't begin until 3-4 hours after ingestion.

5. Carnitine: The main job of this protein (a combination of lysine and methionine to be exact) is to act like a shuttle, transporting fat back and forth into cells. Theories about carnitine allowing glycogen to be spared by making more fat available to exercising muscles have been floating around. Only 4 out of 13 studies show any effects of carnitine enhancing performance. What's more, anything over 6 grams per day is too large a dose and could result in diarrhea. Of the two forms of carnitine (L-carnitine and D-carnitine), only the L-carnitine seems to be safe to use as a supplement.

6. Chromium: Chromium is an essential trace mineral (meaning needed in very small quantities) that has been advertised to stabilize blood sugar levels and increase the making of muscle mass in athletes. Because chromium by itself is not well absorbed, it is often available in the form of chromium picolinate, chromium nicotinate or chromium polynicotinate. Chromium's role in carbohydrate and fat metabolism is related to insulin. Chromium potentiates the action of insulin, so less insulin is required if sufficient chromium (in a usable form) is present. Chromium deficiency can result in high blood sugars, high blood fat levels and high blood cholesterol levels which ultimately lead to cardiac disease. Because we know that strenuous exercise stimulates urinary chromium losses, poor chromium status could result in diminished athletic performance due to the impairment of carbohydrate and fat metabolism. In such cases, adding good sources of chromium to the diet and using a biologically available supplement could return physical performance parameters to normal. If chromium status is already normal, there is no scientific data that indicates chromium supplementation will improve physical performance. Good sources of dietary chromium include mushrooms, oysters and apples with skins. Carbohydrate loading with refined carbohydrates not only results in a chromium-poor diet, but highly refined carbohydrates also stimulate chromium losses. Carbohydrate loading should be done with unrefined carbohydrates, such as whole grains and cereals, legumes, and starchy vegetables.

7. Creatine: Finally! A supplement that's been discovered that isn't considered a gimmick ergogenic. Our bodies produce creatine, but in small amounts; roughly one gram a day. Inside muscle cells, creatine turns into creatine phosphate (CP) which is responsible for giving you the energy for the first few seconds of activity. Repeated studies have shown significant improvement in short bouts of activities that require high levels of strength and power (knee extensions, bench press, running and cycling sprints). However, the studies on endurance activities have generally not reported an ergogenic benefit. Creatine doesn't actually build

muscles. It allows you to work out longer and more intensely without fatiguing as quickly. This means you'll experience faster gains in strength and muscle mass. Available in powder and liquid form, studies report that the maximum muscle storage of creatine is achieved by supplementing 5 grams of creatine monohydrate four times/day for five to six days, followed by a maintenance phase of 2 g/day to replace daily turnover. This is a bit different from the former recommendations of loading on 20-25 grams at once, then dropping to 5 grams per day. Anything more than that after a week of supplementing will not do you any more good, as your muscles can only hold so much creatine. If you're a coffee drinker, caffeine appears to inhibit phosphocreatine resynthesis during recovery from exercise. This will then interfere with any ergogenic effect of creatine. A common side effect reported by athletes is muscle cramping. To avoid this, you must drink plenty of water every day, but it's no guarantee. Recently, studies have shown that for optimal results with creatine you should mix it with some sort of carbohydrate. An example would be a sports drink like Gatorade™. This is for two reasons. One is that the ingestion of carbohydrate will cause the release of insulin, a hormone that promotes glucose uptake into the cell to be used for energy. The other reason is that the carbohydrate itself is a great way to glycogen load. It's like a double-whammy "supercharge" effect when you supplement with creatine/carbohydrate combinations. The caveat: to date, there are no long-term studies on the effects of creatine supplementation and whether or not stopping supplementation after an extended period of time results in muscle loss. It's always a good idea to use caution when taking any supplement, as too much of a good thing can be dangerous.

8. DHEA - Dehydroepiandrosterone: Although many

think this one is a benign and "natural" nutritional supplement that can treat everything from a depressed libido to curing cancer, it's actually a hormone. The most abundant steroid in the bloodstream, and concentrated in the brain, our bodies seem to make less and less DHEA over time. As a result, manufacturers have begun selling DHEA as an "anti-aging" supplement and have done very well in sales. Since DHEA is an anabolic steroid that is naturally secreted by the adrenal glands, it makes sense that men may be enticed to try it to build muscle. But this is not without its side effects when used as a supplement. Enlarged breasts in men and excessive hair growth in women have been documented. Your endocrine (hormone) system is a powerful one and I wouldn't mess with it too much. Bottom line: Don't use it. It's better to be safe, than sorry.

9. Ginseng: Ginseng sales are booming. Touted as an anabolic, antioxidant and an aphrodisiac, ginseng is also known as *panax ginseng*. This comes from the word panacea, meaning "cure-all." Also known to be over 3,000 years old, there are twenty-two different plants that go by the name ginseng. As a result, it can be difficult to figure out which type of ginseng is being used in its various forms such as tea, powders, capsules, extracts, tablets and even ginseng-flavored soft drinks. Although there is no solid evidence that ginseng enhances sexual performance or potency, there is some evidence that it may enhance your ability to cope with mild to moderate stress. In terms of it being considered an ergogenic aid for athletes, studies conclude that ginseng has no significant effect on enhancing performance. Even if ginseng was good for your health, consumers face another hurdle: there's no way to be sure

what's in a ginseng supplement. The amounts of six ginsenosides in 10 different brands of ginseng has been measured and a wide variation was found. The Ginseng labels don't help you tell what's inside. A bottle of Natural Brand Korean labeled "648 mg." had 10 times as much ginsenoside per pill as a bottle of Naturally Korean (a different brand) that was also labeled "648 mg." While findings may not represent each brand nationwide, they are indicative of the brand-to-brand variation a shopper can expect to encounter. Ginsana, the market leader, did appear to be standardized. Single packages from each of three lots had nearly identical ginsenoside profiles.

10. HMB – Beta-hydroxy-beta-methylbutryrate:

It has been suggested that HMB, a metabolic byproduct of leucine (an essential amino acid) acts as an anticatabolic agent. It is thought to prevent muscle breakdown to enhance recovery from exercise. There have been about 3 studies to date that have shown significantly greater strength increases in trained and untrained subjects consuming HMB compared to a placebo, but these ergogenic benefits are equivocal. Additionally, a recent study showed that HMB did not have any adverse effects on health indices in highly trained athletes. However, because very few studies have been conducted and results have been mixed, I would not recommend HMB as a supplement to enhance exercise performance.

11. MCTs – Medium Chain Triglycerides:

MCTs are not as big as the typical fat, LCT or long-chain triglycerides. MCTs are also absorbed and burned differently than LCTs. In fact, MCTs are absorbed directly into the blood system and are burned rather quickly, similar to carbohydrates. When studied, MCTs were found to increase your metabolism. Theoretically, a revved up metabolism would cause you to burn more calories, and thus lose weight. When put to the test again by other researchers, the same results were not able to be duplicated. It can not be concluded that MCTs are "fat-burners," but they may help preserve muscle by preventing its breakdown. Conclusion: stick to the old-fashioned way by exercising more and eating less.

12. Pyruvate: Pyruvate is the end product of glycolysis (a pathway in every cell of our body that creates a small amount of energy anaerobically). If oxygen is available, pyruvate can then go on to enter the aerobic cycles in the cells that create 18 times more energy than glycolysis. If pyruvate is limited, theoretically fatigue results and endurance is limited. Studies that have looked at pyruvate as a supplement show an improvement in aerobic endurance capacity and suggest that this is possibly a result of sparing of muscle glycogen.

The following is a list of additional supplements that are commonly asked about:

Brewer's Yeast

As its name suggests, this brown and bitter substance is most popularly used to infuse beer with its distinctive flavor during the brewing process. But that's not why it's being appreciated as a high-quality dietary supplement. Brewer's yeast is an excellent source of chromium (a mineral that's involved in the regulation of normal blood sugars) and selenium (another mineral known for it's powerful antioxidant functions). In addition, it can be used as a bulking agent to help prevent constipation. That's not all. Brewer's yeast contains high amounts of a substance referred to as SRF (skin respiratory factor) which is involved in skin wound repair. Interestingly, some hemorrhoid ointments' (such as Preparation H) active ingredient includes SRF but I wouldn't apply brewer's yeast directly to an irritated area. Rather, try sprinkling some on your morning cereal. Either way, brewer's yeast is a worthwhile supplement to try as it is not only easy to find in most health food stores but easy on your wallet too. Compared to other dietary supplements, it's inexpensive and nontoxic.

Coenzyme Q_{10} (CoQ_{10})

Also known as ubiquinone, CoQ_{10} gets its name for being ubiquitous, or in virtually every cell of the body. Sellers claim the supplement can "strengthen the heart" and "inhibit the aging process." It's also known to be an antioxidant. The majority of research done on CoQ_{10} is related to its possible links to heart health. The idea is that CoQ_{10} prevents LDLs (the "bad" cholesterol") from oxidation, which is thought to be the first step in the process of plaque buildup that narrows arteries and ultimately leads to cardiovascular disease. The research findings are showing that people with cardiovascular disease are clearly deficient in CoQ_{10}. With all the supplements available today, it's easy to see

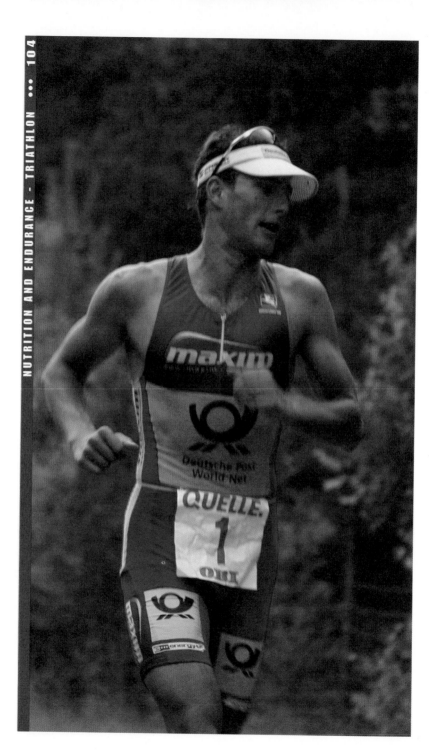

why CoQ$_{10}$ can get lost in the shuffle. However, I think that it should not be scoffed off as another useless product.

Colloidal Minerals

I consider myself an open-minded nutritionist. Although I've been trained to use the "scientific method" in evaluating diets and products, I try not to have unnecessary tunnel vision. But truthfully, colloidal minerals make me cringe. Marketeers claim that they can correct a host of conditions, including cancer, colitis, and even criminal behavior. They go on to say that these solutions of microscopic particles suspended in water are extracted from "special" deposits laid down 10,000 years ago and are better absorbed by the body because of their small size and negative charge.

First, absorption is a function of the body's need, not a mineral's size or electrical charge. Second, high aluminum and silver levels in the body are especially dangerous. These minerals are not merely benign. They are downright unsafe and can even cause a condition characterized by irreversible blue-gray discoloration of the skin known as argyria. Third, the combination of minerals in the capsules are in strange amounts unrelated to human requirements. Finally, supplements that are sold based on testimonials while the "clinical" studies are essentially nonexistent or fabricated are questionable.

If you feel your mineral status warrants extra supplementation, first consider eating more dark green leafy vegetables. If that doesn't satisfy you, try a multivitamin from a reputable nutritional line. Bottom line advice: its better to be safe than sorry. Colloidal minerals offer false hopes at a high price.

Digestive Enzymes

I recently had lunch with one of my "holistic" doctor girlfriends and her mother. As the waitress served us our delightfully prepared quiches and salads, I reached for my fork in anticipation of the pleasure I was about to receive from this familiar favorite. Just before I did though, I looked up only to find my girlfriend casually popping a little capsule that looked like it had some sort of very finely chopped substance in it. Obviously noticing the somewhat puzzled look on my face, she mentioned that she'd begun taking digestive enzymes to help her "assimilate" her nutrients. "Oh, brother", I thought to myself. "Even Susan's been brainwashed. "After all", I thought, "doesn't she know that stuff is useless?" But it seemed like every health care professional I bumped into shortly after that luncheon kept talking about digestive enzymes. It was bothering me. "I'll have to look into this one more carefully", I concluded.

I was surprised to see how much information has been written on this most interesting, often misunderstood supplement. The number of web sites on this topic was especially shocking. My traditional training has taught me that enzymes are involved in every process of the body. Enzymes are catalysts, or transformers. They facilitate chemical reactions without being changed in the process. Enzymes breakdown fats, proteins and carbohydrates into their smaller constituents (glycerol, fatty acids, amino acids and simple sugars), but the enzyme itself remains unchanged. In the body, enzymes can also do the opposite - they can also make smaller molecules join together to form larger ones. The root of much chronic disease and degeneration lies within the impaired ability of proper enzyme activity in the body. Life, itself, could not exist without enzymes. It is commonly known that some foods lose vitamins when cooked or processed. Conversely, raw foods contain just the right amount of enzymes to help break down that particular food.

Why then do such differences in opinions currently exist about the need for digestive enzymes as a supplement? The conventional school of thought teaches that supplemental digestive enzymes are completely unnecessary. The reason? Enzymes are proteins which break down or become "denatured" in the acidic environment of the stomach. Thus, they never even entering the small intestines where they would typically be needed to do the job. The exception: patients with pancreatic insufficiency, often referred to as "malabsorbers," can be given pancreatic enzymes orally. After they enter the mouth and pass through the stomach, they remain intact upon entry into the small intestines, where they then facilitate the nutrient breakdown.

Is it accurate to say that enzymes are useless with that one exception? The answer I found: it used to be. Until manufacturers got a clue and began coating their pills with a substance (enteric coatings) that allows the enzyme to remain intact in the stomach. This enables it to be released in the first part of the intestines (or the duodenum) where its beneficial properties could be reaped. According to the Physicians Desk Reference or PDR, "enteric coatings protect against gastric deactivation and allows delivery of predictable, high levels of biologically active enzymes into the duodenum." The cost of enzymes are now more affordable, as opposed to the cost of enzymes a person with pancreatic disorder would have to purchase. The reason is that some prescription pancreatic enzymes have special – "high tech" delivery systems that give it its attributed two layers of protection. First, the pill has an overall enteric coating for it's first line of protective defense from the stomach acids. Second, inside the encapsulation's preparation, there are hundreds of individual encapsulated microspheres of enterically coated enzymes for further protection.

The pro-enzyme therapy research contends that when raw foods are eaten they basically digest themselves demanding fewer enzymes from the digestive tract to do the job. When cooked, refined or processed foods are eaten, all of the enzymes to digest that food must be supplied by the tissues of the body. One well-known example is that refined foods can promote chromium loss. How so? It appears that the enzymes, B vitamins and chromium must all come from your body's tissue stores in order for the sugar to be metabolized. Eating large quantities of sugar can have the effect of creating a B vitamin and chromium deficiency while simultaneously depleting enzymes.

Plant enzymes containing protease, amylase, lipase and cellulase (the suffix 'ase' refers to an enzyme) are apparently the only enzymes capable of digesting food both in the stomach and small intestine. This is because they work in both acid and alkaline environments. In contrast, pepsin (another digestive enzyme that breaks down protein) works only in the acid environment of the stomach and pancreatin works only in the alkaline environment of the small intestine. In this sense, plant enzymes are more "broad spectrum." An often overlooked point of the advantages of plant enzymes is that they conserve enzymes from the pancreas. Since the pancreas secretes enzymes on demand, the more digested the food is before it reaches the small intestine, the less enzymes the pancreas needs to secrete. Plant enzymes, when taken before a meal, will ensure much further breakdown of food thereby "sparing" enzymes from the pancreas. This puts less of a demand on the pancreas, thus allowing it to perform its other vitally important functions in the body. Plant enzymes should not be viewed as taking a "digestant." They merely put back into the food enzymes similar to those that should be there in the first place. This is the same principle as taking multiple vitamins to help replace those lost.

What is presented here is quite limited in terms of the importance and benefits of digestive enzymes. Hopefully, the attitude towards and understanding of digestive enzymes will eventually change as medical and nutrition science grows out of its infancy.

Fructooligosaccharides (FOS)

This funny sounding word simply refers to a type of a naturally occurring sugar that biochemically is a combination of two simple sugars, fructose (fruit sugar) and sucrose (table sugar). The difference is FOS doesn't behave like simple sugars in the body. It functions more like a soluble fiber, yielding minimal caloric value as it is not really absorbed by your body. Microbial fructooligosaccharides have attracted special attention and is attributing to the expansion of the sugar market by several factors. First, its mass production is not complicated. Second, the sweet taste is very similar to that of sucrose, a traditional sweetener. Since consumption data reflects an increase in consumer demand for safer alternative sweeteners, FOS in the sugar market is expected to rise. So, what's so clever about using this so-called "smart" food ingredient?

Touted to selectively support the survival and growth of intestinal "probiotics" or naturally occurring "good" bacteria (such as acidophilus, bifidus and faecium), FOS seems to show promise of lowering your risk of colon cancer and other diseases. Conversely, pathogenic or "bad" bacteria (including Escherchia coli, Clostridium perfringers and others) have been shown to be unable to use the FOS. Diabetics may benefit from its consumption, as FOS appears to reduce carbohydrate and lipid absorption, thereby normalizing blood glucose and serum lipids. Not a bad added bonus. Natural sources of FOS include a wide variety of edible plants such as banana, garlic, honey, barley, onion, wheat, tomato, rye and brown sugar.

This new functional food is now available in some-health food stores under the brand name Nutraflora™, in a powdered form. Some companies are selling FOS as a nutritional supplement, while others add to their probiotics. Its safety and toxicity is not completely clear, although more and more research is giving it the green light.

Glucosamine and Chondroitin

Two supplements that have received much attention are glucosamine and chondroitin. They are two of the major components of cartilage. In the body, glucosamine is known to stimulate the production of cartilage, improve joint function and reduce pain. Chondroitin helps to draw fluid and nutrients back to the cartilage. If your body is unable to produce the ingredients (such as proteoglycans and collagen) to give cartilage its resilience and shock absorbing functions, a debilitating condition known as osteoarthritis sets in. Theoretically, taking glucosamine and chondroitin supplements can halt, reverse or even cure osteoarthritis. So, is it true? Apparently osteoarthritis can't be cured, but based on the documented results of some well-controlled studies it does seem to help to reduce pain and restore joint function. Fortunately, if you don't experience these results, taking them as supplements is pretty harmless, unlike non-steroidal anti-inflammatory drugs, since they are generally nontoxic. Overall, if osteoarthritis is a problem for you, boning up on glucosamine and chondroitin just may do the trick.

Melatonin

1998's craze. Synthetic versions of this human hormone are said, by the more conservative promoters, to fight insomnia and jet lag. The more daring proponents also claim that it can slow aging, fight disease and enhance one's sex life. Melatonin is produced during the night by the pineal gland located at the base of the brain. Studies have found that taking a fraction of a milligram can hasten sleep. But the evidence is very weak for the claims that melatonin reduces jet lag, can slow aging, fight disease and enhance one's sex life. Several pharmaceutical companies are hoping to turn melatonin into a prescription drug, but you can already buy it in the store. Use of melatonin does have drawbacks. No one knows the right dosage, the interactions with other drugs or the long-term effects. One brand lists extensive cautions, including warnings addressed to people with diabetes, depression, leukemia, epilepsy or autoimmune diseases, and to women who are pregnant or nursing.

Noni Juice

Derived from the Morinda tree, you won't find this product in a health food store, let alone your supermarket. To date, noni juice is only available through a distributor for a hefty $40 per bottle (unless you buy in bulk - you get a $10 break per bottle). But it just might be worth your time and money. Check out this impressive description of what Noni juice has been shown to do for you. Noni juice is yet another anti-inflammatory that appears to enhance the immune system by stimulating what's known as "T—cells," the superstar cells of your immune system that fight off infection and foreign invaders. It also affects your pineal gland which is responsible for regulating your endocrine or hormonal systems. More specifically, it appears to stimulate the release of serotonin and melatonin from the pineal gland (two chemicals that are related to your sense of well-being and sleep cycle, respectively). It's also touted to normalize blood pressure, have antibacterial properties and is considered an antihistaminic agent. From my research, this is only a small list of its alleged properties. Additional functions are related to sophisticated biochemistry and physiology, all of which are beyond the scope of this book. Even though noni juice is expensive, you may want to try this tart tasting drink as it just may provide you with more "bang for your buck" than you realized.

OPCs – Oligomeric Proanthocyanidins (*including Pycnogenol*)

This increasingly popular supplement is another excellent alternative to non-steroidal anti-inflammatory drug use (NSAIDS). NSAIDS are often used for many ailments ranging from stress fractures and pre-menstrual muscle cramping to heart disease and cancer prevention. Although there a few different brand names, such as *pyconogenol*™, a good OPC product will contain pine bark extract, grape seed extract, red wine extract, bilberry extract, and bioflavanoids (citrus extracts). For maximal absorption, it should come in a crystal/powder–like form to be mixed with a small amount of water. Sometimes this is referred to as an "isotonic"

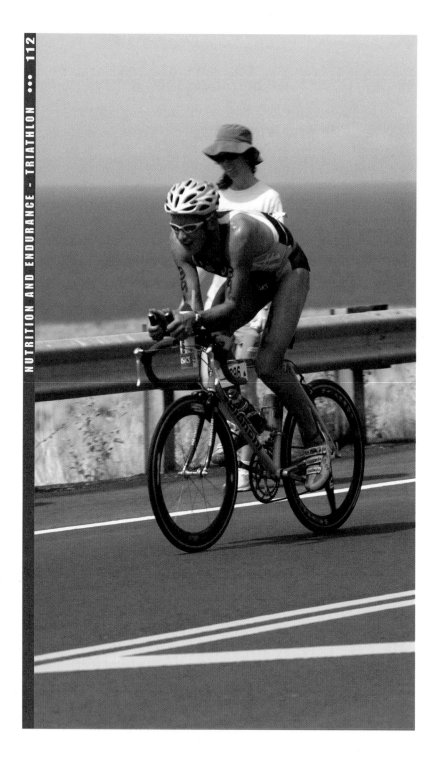

form. It is becoming increasingly evident that these substances are proving to have powerful positive health benefits without the often annoying and undesirable side effects of drug therapy.

Quercetin

What do over 20 million Americans suffer from every year, especially around the arrival of the vernal equinox? If you guessed allergies, you've hit it on the head. With symptoms that span from the all-too-familiar sneezing and runny noses to annoying itchiness and chronic fatigue, allergies can be a nuisance just about any time of the year. Another type of bioflavonoid (one of the classes of phytochemicals) known as quercetin has been identified as being the most potent natural antiallergy substance available. In essence, quercetin seems to have three major beneficial functions. One, it's an anti-inflammatory so the nasal passages, eyes and sinuses don't get irritated. Two, it's an antihistamine. This means it prevents those annoying allergy symptoms like watery eyes and drippy noses by blocking histamines at the site of release. Three, it may have anti-cancer properties. According to the Journal of Anti-Cancer Drugs, quercetin was "shown to inhibit cell cancer lines and oral tumors." Now that's nothing to sneeze at.

Shark Cartilage

Sometimes touted as a glucosamine "wannabe," shark cartilage rose in popularity when the famous "Sharks Don't Get Cancer" literature was released in an attempt to cash in on its most common claim of being an anti-cancer agent. This is mainly because research from the Massachusetts Institute of Technology (MIT) reported that shark cartilage prevents the development of blood vessels that nourish tumors, therefore inhibiting tumor growth. While it may be true that shark cartilage has been studied, the evidence is inconclusive. Fortunately, no serious side effects have been reported to date and there is a great deal of information available on the Internet. Buyer beware: if you are presently on radiation therapy and/or chemotherapy, always consult your physician if you are thinking of abandoning any conventional therapy or even supplementing with alternative remedies.

Tea

One of the oldest beverages, purported to have ingredients with healing properties that range from astringents to antioxidants, tea has only three true varieties. These varieties are black, oolong and green. All come from the same plant. The difference is that black tea is fully fermented, oolong tea is partially fermented and green tea is not fermented at all. While it is the black tea that is rich with the antiseptic properties of tannin, it is the green tea that contains the antioxidant properties (substances that prevent cells from being harmed). It earns this function because green tea contains catechins, a type of phytochemical. It is also a pretty good source of fluoride and may assist in the prevention of dental caries. Now, that's something to smile about.

A word of caution though: many teas have been adulterated with herbs or stimulants (other than caffeine) such as ma huang, a source of ephedra. Manufacturer's often sell them for weight control or constipation under names such as cowboy tea, desert herb, mormon tea, popotillio and squaw tea. Ephedra (banned by the US FDA in January 2004) is a dangerous stimulant which proves that just because a substance is "natural" it can be just as potent as drug use. In fact, several serious incidents have been reported (including death). You may have seen "diet teas" available that claim to be the "natural" way to lose weight. Senna, the main ingredient in these products, is really a herbal laxative that promotes water loss. The problem is that it stimulates the large intestines, which can also result in dehydration, nausea and even extreme diarrhea. Whether in the form of tea or a plain ol' pill, laxatives should only be taken sparingly and on the advice of a physician. The bottom line: don't mess with laxatives. They are addictive substances that will get you in trouble with your bowel movements and your hydration status if you abuse them.

Brain Foods: Bogus or Pure Pabulum?

As the number of Internet users grows exponentially in this information age, so have the number of pabular supplements claiming to "feed your head" or "think fast." You won't have to rack your brains too hard as this next short section serves to demystify these cognitive claims of improved memory and intelligence.

Choline/Lecithin

Sometimes confused as a B-vitamin, choline is a non-essential amino acid is used to make other important substances such as acetylcholine and lecithin. (Recall from Chapter 1 that a non-essential amino acid simply means that your body can manufacture it from another substance, thus it is not "essential" or required to receive it from dietary sources). In this case choline is made from the essential amino acid methionine. As for these other technical sounding terms, acetylcholine is a neurotransmitter or "brain messenger" released by the part of our nervous system that's responsible for activities such as resting and digesting. Compared to the gas and brake pedal of an automobile, it can be likened to the brake pedal that stops or slows a car down. Without it, your brain's "wiring" system would get all wacky and your thoughts would become confused. It now appears that extra amounts of choline may be helpful in the treatment of Alzheimer's disease, but does not seem to improve the mental functioning of otherwise healthy individuals. Choline, no doubt, is needed by the body to perform important brain related functions, but natural choline deficiencies don't exist since we get enough choline in our diets. In addition, supplementing on choline may cause nausea, vomiting dizziness and depression.

Lecithin is a combination of a fat and choline stuck together. Both nature and the food industry use lecithin as an emulsifier to combine two ingredients that do not ordinarily mix, such as oil and water.

DHA (docosahexanoic acid)
See Chapter 6 – Fat Matters

Flaxseed

This popular light brown seed resembles the sesame seed in size and shape and has a pleasant nutty flavor. Flaxseed is an excellent source of protein and fiber, while its oil is rich with linolenic acid (the much touted Omega-3 fatty acid). It's also high in the group of phytochemicals called lignans that have anticancer effects. The biggest concern about flaxseed oil is how quickly it can go rancid. Proper preparation and storage are the key to keeping it from spoiling. For example, it's best to buy flaxseed whole and then grind it up as needed. Since light and heat will affect it too, keep it refrigerated in opaque bottles and don't cook with it. Avoid buying the "cold-pressed" oils as this modification robs it of its health benefits. Taking these measures can mean the difference between benefiting versus harming yourself with food. Overall, flaxseed is a delicious and healthy food supplement to try. Did you know that you cannot only eat this stuff, you can wear it too! Flax is the source of linen fiber. Talk about getting your money's worth!

Ginkgo Biloba

Ginkgo falls under this category because of its use for "brain-related" things like enhancing memory or even treating patients with Alzheimer's disease. This funny sounding herb has been getting thumbs up for easing symptoms related to dementia, senility, memory loss, dizziness, headache, tinnitus (ringing in the ears) and muscle cramping. That's because it appears to increase the flow of blood and oxygen to the brain by acting as a vasodilater. For the elderly, that translates into treatment for Alzheimer's disease. Gingko is most commonly used in an extract form but can be found in tea leaves, tinctures and tablets.

Super blue-green algae (SBGA)

This supplement, sometimes called spirulina, has been categorized as everything from "pond scum" to "brain food." Once again, it is another substance that relies on mostly anecdotal evidence rather than scientific support to justify its claims. Some claims include increased stamina, improved mental clarity, better digestion and an improved attitude. This so-called "magical" algae is probably more accurately described as a "monster" algae, as serious side effects have been reported (nausea, vomiting, headaches, dizziness and even uterine bleeding). Even so, SBGA is big business, as sales in 1995 approached an estimated $8 million. Not bad for pond scum.

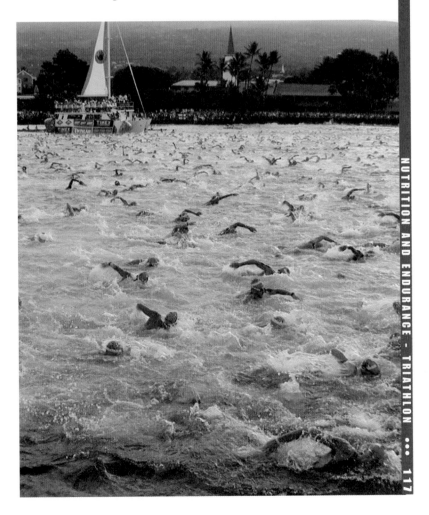

Superstar Nutrients

With all the emphasis on non-traditional nutrients that we're just learning about, let's not forget about the vital nutrients that we've known from the beginning have been vital to our health. Focusing on only the most raved about nutrients, this section will give you the latest scoop on the "superstars" of nutrition today.

Antioxidants

As trendy as they seem to be, there's nothing new about the known existence of antioxidants. They are crucial in the prevention of diseases and preservation of good health. But what exactly are antioxidants anyway? A textbook definition would tell you that antioxidants are substances that donate electrons to another substance. In essence, antioxidants are nutrients that will happily protect other nutrients from being attacked or damaged by allowing itself to get oxidized instead. Wow. What a martyr.

The following nutrients are examples of a few antioxidants:

Beta-carotene
Beta-carotene, involved in vision function, is a precursor to and plant form of vitamin A. It is considered the most important of the carotenoids. Carotenoids, a pigment commonly found in some yellow and orange plants such as carrots, pumpkin, sweet potatoes, canteloupe, and winter squash, are among the best known phytochemicals.

Vitamin C
Ever wonder why your mother told you to pour a little orange juice or lemon juice on a fruit salad so it wouldn't turn brown? Orange and lemon juice contain vitamin C which will preserve the fruit thanks to the antioxidant properties. Probably one of the

most controversial vitamins in terms of ideal dosage, (scientists argue needs range between 75 mg to 10,000 mg per day!), vitamin C is a well known antioxidant. In fact, it ranks right up there with chicken soup for combating the common cold. Also known as ascorbic acid, it has a number of other functions including connective tissue development and maintenance, wound healing and hormone synthesis.

Vitamin E

It is amazing how far this valuable fat-soluble vitamin has come. A once rather neglected vitamin, it is now known that vitamin E plays a profound role in heart health. The reason is because not only is vitamin E a known antioxidant, it also functions as an anticoagulant (anticoagulants reduce the blood's ability to clot, thus reducing the risk of clot-related stroke and heart attack). Daily supplementation of up to 800 IUs (international units) may reduce the risk of non-fatal heart attacks. Be sure to look for "natural" vitamin E in the form of "mixed tocopherols." Good food sources of vitamin E include wheat germ, vegetable oils, nuts and seeds.

Selenium

A mineral that works with vitamin E, selenium is a powerful antioxidant that's found in a variety of both animal and plant sources. If it's so widespread, is supplementing with selenium necessary? Some argue that the soil of the United States' farmlands have been depleted of many precious minerals, especially selenium. As a result, they claim that neither our farm animals who rely on plant life grown in this soil, nor the actual plant food itself ends up with much selenium to offer. The truth is that the problem of "soil depletion" varies from one area to another, so it's very difficult to know the nature of the soils at any given time. People should be eating more fruits and vegetables anyway, but if this is a problem for you, a good multivitamin/ mineral supplement should do the trick.

Zinc

It used to be that when you thought of a nutrient that was associated with easing the symptoms of the common cold, you thought of vitamin C. Then, in 1996, along came the famous Cleveland Clinic study on zinc and it's cold-fighting potential. The results were strong enough to pave the way for yet another nutrient to be packaged and marketed as the "cold season dietary supplement." In order for zinc to do the job, it must be taken in a form that is unbound to other substances such as sorbitol, mannitol or citric acid, common additives for flavor enhancement. That's because ingredients added to zinc will prevent it from being absorbed in the mouth where zinc is needed for colds. Zinc attached to gluconate seems to be the best form as compared to zinc aspartate or zinc citrate which are inactive in the mouth. Therefore, zinc lozenges are more effective than zinc pills. It's best that you don't chew the lozenge. Instead, suck on it to help keep it in your mouth for as long as possible. That's because zinc works on nasal passageways, where it prevents a virus from attacking in the first place. Finally, because zinc competes for the same enzymes in your body as other important nutrients such as copper, make sure your zeal for zinc is within reason. Too much could lead to a copper deficiency.

Other Nutrients in the Limelight

Calcium – Just the skeletal bone facts

Although not a mineral that is exclusive to women's health, calcium nutrition is of great concern for a vast majority of females. And it should be. Adequate calcium intake throughout life can help prevent osteoporosis, a debilitating disease of bone demineralization. Many wonder why routine blood tests never show any calcium deficiency and suddenly, a woman falls and breaks her hip, only to be told that she has osteoporosis! The answer is that your bones are like a "bank" of calcium. If you don't get your calcium from your diet (or supplements) your body will meet its first priority and withdraw calcium from your bones to deposit into the blood to maintain its tightly regulated calcium levels. When you do get calcium from your diet, it will first take what it needs for your bodily functions that require calcium and then deposit back into the bone. Pretty impressive, eh?

The current calcium RDA for women over age 25 is 1000mg/day; however, many experts recommend a higher intake level (1000-1500 mg/day). This level can be met with dairy products, canned fish containing bones, tofu, or certain greens. Calcium is a mineral that is generally found bound to a "salt." The salt portion of a supplement is simply excreted by the body. So when reading labels, be sure to look for the amount of elemental calcium, that is, calcium that's actually available for absorption by the body. There are various types of calcium "salts", some of the more popular preparations being calcium carbonate (i.e. Tums, Caltrate, Os-Cal), and calcium citrate (Citri-Cal). Calcium carbonate is the most concentrated and least expensive calcium source (40% calcium) so that taking this preparation enables women to consume fewer or smaller-size tablets. It should be taken with meals to ensure maximum absorption. Calcium citrate, however, is slightly better absorbed than calcium carbonate, but contains less elemental calcium per tablet, requiring more tablets to be taken daily. In addition, calcium citrate supplements are usually more expensive than other types of calcium supplements and should be taken on an empty stomach.

Absorption of calcium is most efficient in single doses of 500 mg or less, and a divided dose regimen results in greater absorption of a supplement than once-a-day dosing. Some calcium preparations, such as the natural product bone meal and dolomite, should be avoided as they may be contaminated with lead and other heavy metals.

There are reasons to be cautious with calcium supplementation. It may cause constipation, and excess calcium (> 2000 mg) may lead to kidney stones. Although calcium supplements are available over-the-counter, they should only be ingested in high doses with a physician's evaluation and concurrence.

Folic Acid

It's scary to know that the deficiency of only one vitamin, while pregnant, can be the cause of robbing a newborn's chance at health. Folic acid, a well known B-vitamin, is crucial to the production of the genetic makeup and growth of each cell. As of January 1st, 1998, manufacturers have been required to add folic acid to all enriched wheat products, including flour, bread, rice and pasta. Amazingly, the recommended dietary intake is a miniscule 400 micrograms (that's 1/1000 of a milligram!), yet without it, horrible neural tube defects such as spina bifida (where the spinal column fails to close during fetal development) or anencephaly (where the brain does not completely develop) can result. Adding folic acid to the food supply will provide an additional 100 micrograms to that.

The Homocysteine-Heart Connection

The health benefits gained by adding folic acid to refined wheat products may be killing two birds with one stone. How so? It appears that folic acid helps decrease the risk of heart disease and stroke. It does this indirectly by reducing abnormally high levels of homocysteine, an amino acid which is the culprit behind the heightened risk of heart disease and stroke. Whether the fortified folic acid will make a difference is yet to be seen. Either way, it's always a good idea to continue to try to get as much folic acid from your food and consider taking a multivitamin/mineral supplement to help balance it with other important nutrients. Careful though; getting more than 1,500 micrograms may mask a vitamin B12 deficiency, if one exists. When in doubt, be sure to check with your doctor.

Iron

Ever hear complaints of "tired blood?" If you have, that should give you a clue as to one of the many functions of iron. Iron is found in a substance called hemoglobin, which acts like a "taxi cab" driving iron to all of the cells of the body to help accept, carry and release oxygen. Iron is also required by enzymes involved in the making of amino acids, hormones and neurotransmitters. If you are deficient in iron, your body's ability to carry oxygen can become impaired. This can result in iron deficiency anemia which leaves you feeling exceptionally tired. Iron has a knack of switching back and forth between two states: its reduced and its oxidized state. Iron in the reduced state (also referred to as ferrous iron) is better absorbed than iron in it's oxidized state (ferric iron). Its absorption is influenced either positively or negatively by many factors. For example, vitamin C, an antioxidant, will increase iron absorption in the intestines. Knowing how an antioxidant works, this makes sense. Vitamin C prevents iron from shifting to its oxidized form by allowing itself to get oxidized instead. This keeps it in its reduced state. Since supplemental iron is already in the form of ferrous iron (the better absorbed state), taking vitamin C with it will not increase its absorption further. The interesting dichotomy of iron is that, worldwide, iron deficiency is the most common nutrient deficiency. If affects an estimated 15 percent of the world's population, with the highest prevalence in developing countries. Young children and pregnant women are especially vulnerable. But in the United States, an estimated 10 percent of the population is in positive iron balance (versus neutral or negative balance), with 1 percent having iron overload. Iron overload is more common in men than in women and is twice as prevalent among men as is iron deficiency. Supplementing with iron should only be done under the direction of a physician, as an iron overdose is the leading cause of poisoning deaths in children. Symptoms of iron toxicity include constipation, nausea, vomiting, a rapid heartbeat, dizziness, shock and confusion.

Magnesium

Involved in over 300 of the body's enzymes systems, only about one ounce of magnesium is present in the body of a 130-pound person. Together with calcium, magnesium is involved in muscle contraction and blood clotting: calcium promotes the processes, whereas magnesium inhibits them. This dynamic interaction between the two minerals helps regulate the functioning of the lungs. Magnesium helps prevent dental caries by holding calcium in tooth enamel and also supports the normal functioning of the immune system. Magnesium has been receiving attention for its role in the maintenance of normal blood pressure as well.

However, there are two distinct kinds of hypertensive patients who are responsive to nutritional supplementation. The magnesium-responsive high blood pressure is one in which the patient is

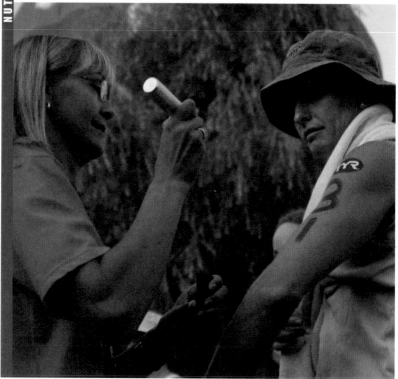

not salt-sensitive and has an elevated or high normal blood level of the kidney hormone, renin. Give these hypertensive individuals magnesium supplements and their blood pressure will come down. The other group includes those individuals who are salt-sensitive (about 20% of all hypertensive patients) and have normal or low normal levels of blood renin. Give these people calcium supplements and their blood pressure will come down. Additionally, some researchers argue that supplementing with therapeutic doses of both magnesium and vitamin B6, may bring extremely painful kidney stone attacks to a complete stop (most recurring kidney stones are composed of calcium oxalate).

Is it More Beneficial to Crush Vitamins?

No. It is not beneficial to crush vitamins. First, if you do so you are exposing the vitamin to oxygen and light, both of which will destroy most vitamins. Minerals, on the other hand, are indestructible elements, so you can't really "crush" them anyway. Second, many vitamins are now "time-released." They are designed with an enteric coating on the pill that will withstand the acid of the stomach and instead will dissolve/react to the more alkaline/neutral pH of the small intestines. This is where nutrients are optimally absorbed. (When food from the stomach enters the small intestines the sodium bicarbonate in the pancreatic juices will alter the acidic food from the stomach to make it all the more neutrally/slightly alkaline).

If Two Is Good, Four Must Be Better. Right?

Ever hear of the bell shaped curve? All it means, in this context, is that there is an optimal range of intake for all nutrients. Although that range may differ from one to the next, taking too little or too much is inappropriate. At one point, the advantages or "returns" from the nutrient you consume begins to diminish, (hence, the economic term, "the point of diminishing returns"). This occurs by decreasing absorption rates as a result of an overload of nutrients. It's really a defense mechanism if you think about it. Your body tries to protect you from toxic doses by preventing it from absorbing the vitamin. Another way your body protects you from overdosing is by increasing the rate at which you excrete nutrients. For example, water-soluble vitamins (B-complex and C) are simply excreted in the urine when you consume more than your body needs. If you continue to bombard your body with these very high doses of nutrients (also called pharmacological doses) there is only so much your body can do to protect you and symptoms of toxicity could appear. Be safe and stick with the RDI (recommended dietary intake) as a starting point. Then with the approval of a health care provider, such as a doctor or registered dietitian, titrate as it's deemed necessary.

A Final Word

So, is there really such a thing as a panacea or a single "cure-all" food? If you ask me, there never was and there never will be. If there was, Mother Nature would not have blessed us with the abundance and gorgeous variety in taste, texture, aroma and color of food. The key is to partake of this variety of healthy food with an attitude of gratitude, moderation and balance.

Although this is truly an exciting and unique time to live, consider that medicine is just coming out of its infancy. Today we learn about things like noni juice, OPCs or digestive enzymes. Tomorrow we'll learn about even bigger, better, more potent nutrients. Food scientists are just beginning to discover and unravel the mysteries and miracles of food as we knew it. Aromas and colors of fruits and vegetables were once considered benign and useless. Today, we know these substances have been identified as power phytochemicals and are considered to greatly improve and maintain health. As our technology and collective health consciousness grows, the keys to unlocking the secrets of good health and longevity will as well. As far as conventional medicine is concerned, it undoubtedly plays an extremely important role in health care. In this swiftly growing day and age of alternative treatment, one can not mitigate the fact that a healthy perspective and appropriate balance of these two worlds must be achieved in order to optimize your level of wellness.

Section III – Key Ideas

It's always best to get your nutrients from food rather than a pill, but backup from supplements may be worthwhile. A good multivitamin should include additional phytochemicals and herbs. Depending on the need, extra Vt. E, Vt. C, calcium, chromium, omega-3 fatty acids or glucasomine/chondroitin might be beneficial. Remember, these supplements are not drugs, so you may not feel the effects of this sort of supplementation immediately, as it may take a while for it to "kick in."

Did you know that according to the Nutrition Business Journal, supplement sales have been steadily increasing and reached $16.7 billion in the year 2000?

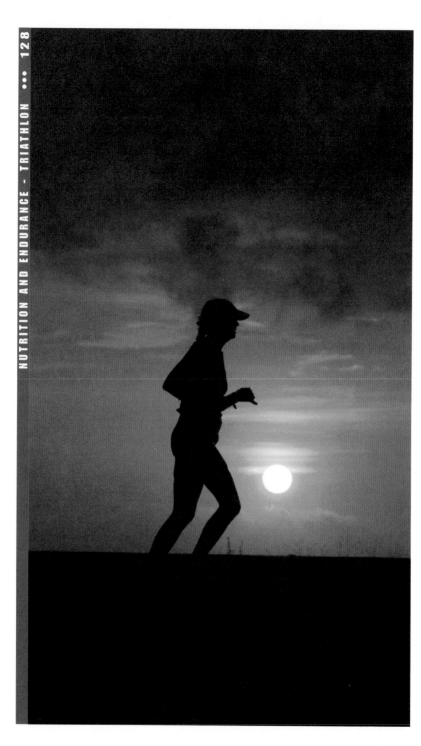

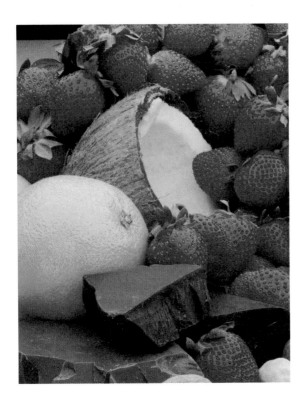

Appendices

- Related Organizations, Associations and Institutes

- Health, Nutrition and Fitness related Newsletters

- Reliable Internet Resources

- References

- Daily Food Journal

- Vitamin and Mineral Summary Table

Related Organizations, Associations and Institutes

Aerobics and Fitness Association of America (AFAA)
15250 Ventura Blvd., Suite 200
Sherman Oaks, CA 91403
800-233-4886
Magazine: American Fitness
www.afaa.com

American Anorexia/Bulimia Association
c/o Regents Hospital
425 East 61st St., 6th floor
New York, NY 10021
212-981-8686

American Cancer Society
1599 Clifton Road NE
Atlanta, GA 30329
800-227-2345
www.cancer.org

American College of Sports Medicine
PO Box 1440
Indianapolis, IN 46206-1440
317-637-9200
Journal: Medicine and Science in Sports and Exercise
www.acsm.org/sportsmed

American Council on Exercise (ACE)
PO Box 910449
San Diego, CA 92191-0449
619-535-8227
www.acefitness.org

American Diabetes Association, Communications Department
1660 Duke St.
Alexandria, VA 22314
800-232-3472 ext. 290
Journals: Diabetes, Diabetes Care, Diabetes Review, and Diabetes
Forecast
www.diabetes.org

American Dietetics Association, National Center for Nutrition and
Dietetics
216 W. Jackson Boulevard
Chicago, IL 60606-6995
800-366-1655
Journal: Journal of the American Dietetic Association
www.eatright.org

American Heart Association, National Center
7272 Greenville Ave.
Dallas, TX 75231
800-242-8721
www.amhrt.org

American Running and Fitness Association
4405 East West Highway, Suite 405
Bethesda, MD 20814
301-913-9517
Newsletter: Running and FitNews
www.arfa.org

Center for Science in the Public Interest
1875 Connecticut Ave. NW, Suite 300
Washington, DC 20009-5728
202-332-9110
Newsletter: Nutrition Action Health Letter
E-mail address: cspi@cspi.net.org

Food and Nutrition Information Center, National Agricultural Library
USDA Room 304, 10301 Baltimore Blvd.
Beltsville, MD 20705-2351
301-504-5719

Gatorade Sports Science Institute
PO Box 9005
Chicago IL 60604
312-222-7704
Newsletter: Sports Science Exchange
www.gssiweb.com

IDEA, The International Association for Fitness Professionals
6190 Cornerstone Court East, Suite 204
San Diego, CA 92121
619-535-8979

International Food Information Council Foundation
1100 Connecticut Avenue, NW, Suite 430
Washington, DC 20036
202-296-6540
E-mail address: foodinfo@ific.health.org

National Center Against Health Fraud (NCAHF)
PO Box 1276
Loma Linda, CA 92354
909-824-4690
Newsletter: NCAHF Newsletter
www.primenet.com/ ~ ncahf/

National Dairy Council, O'Hare International Center
10255 West Higgins Road, Suite 900
Rosemont, IL 60018
708-803-2000
Newsletter: Dairy Council Digest

National Strength and Conditioning Association
PO Box 38909
Colorado Springs, CO 80934
719-632-6722
Journal of Strength and Conditioning Research and Strength and Conditioning

President's Council on Physical Fitness and Sports
701 Pennsylvania Avenue NW, Suite 250
Washington, DC 20004
202-272-3421

Vegetarian Resource Group
PO Box 1463
Baltimore, MD 21203
410-366-8343
Magazine: The Vegetarian Journal

Women's Sports Foundation
Eisenhower Park
East Meadow, NY 11554
800-227-3988
Newsletter: Women's Sports Experience

Eating Disorders Review, Raven Press
1185 Avenue of the Americas
New York, NY 10036
800-853-2478

Environmental Nutrition
PO Box 420451
Palm Coast, FL 32142-0300
800-829-5384

Harvard Medical School Health Letter
PO Box 420300
Palm Coast, FL 32142-0300
800-829-9045

Nutrition & the MD, Raven Press
1185 Avenue of the Americas, New York, NY 10036
800-853-2478

Penn State Sports Medicine Newsletter
PO Box 6568
Syracuse, NY 1317-9976
800-825-0061

Sports Medicine Digest, Raven Press
1185 Avenue of the Americas, New York, NY 10036
800-853-2478

Tufts University Diet and Nutrition Letter
PO Box 57857
Boulder, CO 80322-7857
800-274-7581
www.healthletter.tufts.edu

Reliable Internet Resources

A quick note about dealing with health related web-sites: Although it is easier now than ever to access information through the Internet, the implications are a mixed bag. The Internet can increase patient awareness and save lives, but it can also waste time, give a patient false hopes and even endanger lives. Virtually anyone can run a health-related web page, and there is no verification of online information. Many commercial and governmental Internet sites can be extremely helpful. However, for all the valid information online, there is also a great deal that is questionable. While the distinction can be made by a discerning eye, patients can often be desperate. In time, as the bad information is filtered away, the Internet should be able to take on an even greater role in medicine and health. Right now the Internet is like a huge gusher of an oil well. The refineries are just beginning to be built. So, if you find yourself throwing your arms up in despair after learning about the plethora of health related web sites out there, try using some of the following sites. I especially like the Tufts Nutrition Navigator site whose job it is to comb through all those sites for you and tell you which ones are worth your time and which ones to avoid.

1. Ironman Triathlon:
    www.ironmanlive.com

2. Department of Health and Human Services Healthfinder:
    www.healthfinder.gov

3. Health on the Net Foundation:
    www.hon.ch.org

4. International Food Information Council:
    www.ificinfo.health.org

5. National Council Against Health Fraud, Inc:
    www.ncahf.org

6. National Institutes of Health:
    www.nih.gov

7. PubMed:
    www.ncbi.nlm.nih.gov/PubMed/

8. Tufts Nutrition Navigator:
    www.navigator.tufts.edu

9. American Botanical Council:
    www.herbalgram.org

10. The Herb Research Foundation:
    www.herbs.org

11. Exercise Physiology Club on the Internet:
    www.exer-phys-club.com

12. Dietetics Online – Professional Networking Organization:
    www.dietetics.com

13. USDA Center for Nutrition Policy and Promotion:
    www.usda.gov/fcs/cnpp.html

14. Vegetarian Resource Group (VRG):
    www.envirolink.org/arrs/VRG/home

15. USDA Food and Nutrition Information Center:
    www.nal.usda.gov/fnic

References

Applegate, L. 1991. Nutritional considerations of ultradistance performance. *Intl. J. Sports Nutrition* 1(1): 3-27.

Blom PCS, et al. 1987. Effect of differenct post-exercise sugar diets on the rate of muscle glycogen synthesis. *Med. Sci. Sports Ex.* 19: 491-496.

Browns, F., et al. 1989. Eating, drinking, and cycling: a controlled Tour de France simulation study. Part I and II. *Int. J. Sport Med.* 10:/S32-S48 (Suppl).

Castel, LM. 1997. The effects of oral glutamine supplementation on athletes after prolonged exhaustive exercise. *Nutrition.* 13: 738-742.

Costill, DL. 1985. Carbohydrate nutrition before, during, and after exercise. *Fed Proc.* 44: 364-368.

The Health Professionals Guide to Popular Dietary Supplements, 2nd ed. Allison Sarubin Fragakis, MS, RD. The American Dietetic Association, 2003.

Kritchevsky D., et al. 1980. Influence of type of carbohydrate on atherosclerosis. *Am J. Clin. Nutr.* 33: 1869.

McArdle, Katch and Katch. Essentials of Exercise Physiology. Williams & Wilkins, 1994.

Noakes, TD. et al. 1993, Fluid replacement during exercise. *Exerc. Sports Sci. rev.* 21: 297-330.

Optimum Sports Nutrition - Michael Colgan, Ph. D. Advanced Research Press, 1993.

Power Eating - Susan M Kleiner, Ph. D., RD. Human Kinetics, 1998.

Rohde, T. 1996. The immune systems and serum glutamine during a triathlon. *Eur. J. Appl. Physiol.* 74: 428-434.

Sports Nutrition Guidebook, 2nd ed - Nancy Clark, MS, RD. Human Kinetics, 1997.

The Ultimate Sports Nutrition Handbook - Ellen Coleman, MPH, MA, RD and Suzanne Nelson Steen, D. Sc., RD. Bull Publishing, 1996.

Zawadzki, KM. 1992. Carbohydrates-protein complex increase the rate of muscle glycogen storage after exercise. *J. Appl. Physiol.* 72(5): 1854-1859.

VITAMIN AND MINERAL SUMMARY TABLE OF RECOMMENDED DIETARY ALLOWANCES (RDA) AND BASIC BIOLOGICAL FUNCTIONS

(note: mcg = micrograms, mg = milligrams)

VITAMIN	RDA	FUNCTION
Fat-Soluble:		
Vitamin A	900 mcg RE or 5000 IU	~ maintenance of healthy skin, eyes, bones, hair and teeth
Vitamin D	5-10 mcg or 400 IU	~ assists in the absorption and metabolism of calcium and phosphorus for strong bones and teeth
Vitamin E	15 mg α-TE*	~ as an antioxidant, helps protect cell membranes, lipoproteins, fats and vitamin A from destructive oxidation
Vitamin K	120 mcg	~ important in blood clotting; helps to regulate blood calcium
Water-Soluble:		
Thiamin (B1)	1.2 mg/day	~ involved in energy metabolism; supports normal appetite and nerve function
Riboflavin (B2)	1.3 mg/day	~ involved in energy metabolism: supports normal vision and skin health
Niacin	16 NE**/day	~ involved in energy metabolism: supports health of skin, nervous system and digestive system
Biotin	30 mcg/day	~ involved in energy metabolism, fat synthesis, protein synthesis, and carbohydrate synthesis
Pantothenic Acid	5 mg/day	~ involved in energy metabolism (specifically part of coenzyme A)
Pyridoxine (B6)	1.3 mg/day	~ used in protein and fat metabolism; helps to make red blood cells
Folic acid (folate)	400 mcg/day	~ involved in genetic makeup of cells; especially important for newly forming cells

*   *α-tocopherol equivalents*

**   *niacin equivalents*

VITAMIN AND MINERAL SUMMARY TABLE
OF RECOMMENDED DIETARY ALLOWANCES (RDA) AND
BASIC BIOLOGICAL FUNCTIONS

(note: mcg = micrograms, mg = milligrams)

VITAMIN	RDA	FUNCTION
Cobalamin (B12)	2.4 mcg/day	~ involved in the making of new cells, helps to maintain nerve cells, helps to break down some fats and proteins
Ascorbic acid (Vt. C)	90 mg/day	~ antioxidant, strengthens resistance to infection, helps keep iron in the form that's best absorbed; thyroxin synthesis, strengthens blood vessel walls, forms scar tissue, provides the matrix for bone growth, involved in protein metabolism

MINERAL	RDA	FUNCTION

Major Minerals

Sodium	500 mg/day	~ assists in nerve impulse transmission and muscle contraction; an electrolyte that maintains normal fluid and electrolyte balance
Chloride	750 mg/day	~ part of HCL found in the stomach, necessary for proper digestion; an electrolyte that maintains normal fluid and electrolyte balance
Potassium	2000 mg/day	~ facilitates many reactions; supports cell integrity; assists in nerve impulse transmission and muscle contractions; an electrolyte that maintains normal fluid and electrolyte balance
Calcium	1000 mg/day	~ involved in muscle contraction and relaxation, blood clotting, blood pressure, nerve functioning, immune defenses; the main mineral of teeth and bones

VITAMIN AND MINERAL SUMMARY TABLE
OF RECOMMENDED DIETARY ALLOWANCES (RDA) AND
BASIC BIOLOGICAL FUNCTIONS
(note: mcg = micrograms, mg = milligrams)

MINERAL	RDA	FUNCTION
Phosphorus	700 mg/day	~ important in genetic material, part of phospholipids, used in energy transfer and in buffer systems that maintain acid-base balance, a main mineral of teeth and bones
Magnesium	400 mg/day	~ involved in the building of protein, bone mineralization, enzyme action, nerve impulse transmission, normal muscular contraction, maintenance of teeth, and functioning of immune system
Sulfer	unestablished	~ part of the B-vitamins, thiamin and biotin, and the hormone insulin, as part of proteins, stabilizes their shape by forming disulfide bridges between them

Trace Minerals:

Iron	18 mg/day	~ part of the protein, hemoglobin, in the blood, which carries oxygen throughout the body; part of the protein, myoglobin in the muscles, which makes oxygen available for muscle contraction; necessary for the calories to be metabolized
Zinc	11 mg/day	~ involved in wound healing; immune reactions, transport of vitamin A, taste perception, the making of sperm, the normal development of the fetus, a part of many enzymes, associated with the hormone insulin, and involved in making genetic material and proteins
Iodine	150 mcg/day	~ a part of two thyroid hormones that help regulate metabolic rate, growth and development

VITAMIN AND MINERAL SUMMARY TABLE
OF RECOMMENDED DIETARY ALLOWANCES (RDA) AND
BASIC BIOLOGICAL FUNCTIONS

(note: mcg = micrograms, mg = milligrams)

MINERAL	RDA	FUNCTION
Selenium	55 mcg/day	~ an antioxidant that works with vitamin E to protect body compounds from oxidation
Copper	900 mcg/day	~ a part of several enzymes; necessary for the absorption and use of iron in the making of hemoglobin
Manganese	2.3 mg/day	~ acts as a facilitator, with enzymes of various cell processes
Fluoride	3.8 mg/day	~ involved in the making of teeth and bones; helps to prevent dental caries
Chromium	35 mcg/day	~ part of GTF, glucose tolerance factor, that assists insulin to control blood sugar levels
Molybdenum	45 mcg/day	~ acts as a facilitator, with enzymes of various cell processes

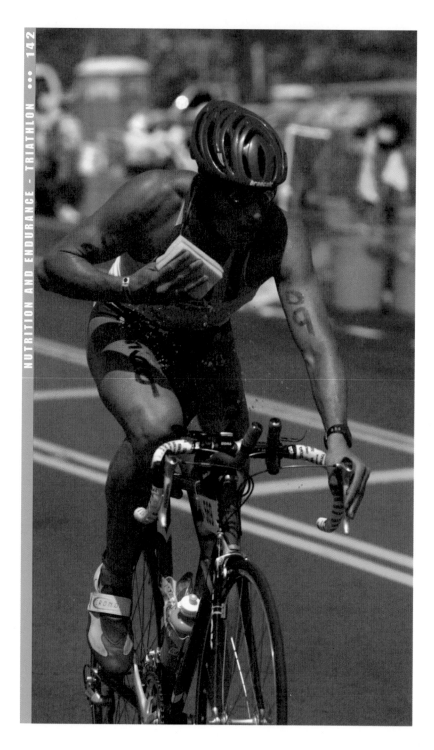

MODEL FOR A DAILY FOOD JOURNAL

TIME	FOOD HOW PREPARED	AMOUNT CONSUMED	ACTIVITY & FEELINGS*	HUNGER LEVEL*

*activity: record the associated activity. For example: watching tv, driving, at table, on the phone

*feelings: record how you felt. For example: were you bored, upset, stressed, excited, tired?

*hunger level: record how hungry or full you were BEFORE you ate. Use a scale from 1-10.

A 1 represents extreme hunger. A 10 represents extreme feeling of fullness

Photo & Illustration Credits: